Before Aspirin
&
Other Things

Before Aspirin & Other Things

Rev. Joseph E. Fulford

iUniverse, Inc.
New York Lincoln Shanghai

Before Aspirin & Other Things

Copyright © 2006 by Joseph E. Fulford

iUniverse books may be ordered through booksellers or by contacting:

iUniverse
2021 Pine Lake Road, Suite 100
Lincoln, NE 68512
www.iuniverse.com
1-800-Authors (1-800-288-4677)

All biblical references came from:
The Kings James Version of the Holy Bible, Copyright 1976 by Thomas Nelson, Inc.
The New King James Version, New Testament, Copyright 1979 by Thomas Nelson, Inc.

ISBN-13: 978-0-595-41608-0 (pbk)
ISBN-13: 978-0-595-85957-3 (ebk)
ISBN-10: 0-595-41608-X (pbk)
ISBN-10: 0-595-85957-7 (ebk)

Printed in the United States of America

Contents

THE NOSE AND THE COFFIN

It was winter and I was eight years old when my uncle died. His body lay on the bed under a white sheet at the farm house. We all went. It was then I experienced my first serious thoughts about death and what follows.

Small gatherings of people stood around the dirt yard and on the porch engaged in quiet conversation. My widowed aunt sat in the parlor in her black taffeta dress. Family members and friends met her with hugs and weeping.

Outside, a still sadness had settled over the cold, sunbright day. At the corner of the yard the coffin-maker fashioned my uncle's casket on two sawhorses. The tap-tap-tap of his hammer on eight-penny nails gave dispirited rhythm to the downcast feeling I already felt in the cold air.

Then, when my uncle's body was placed in the pine pall, a serious flaw was detected. It seemed the carpenter had not given due consideration to my uncle's long, sharp nose when calculating the depth of the coffin. And when he was laid in, it became painfully obvious that the lid would flatten his nose when closed.

Promptly, there issued from my aunt and her sisters such a tirade of dissatisfaction that the craftsman was more than willing to correct the defect.

"O, yes," he said. "I can fix that easily—no problem."

He lifted my uncle's body a little and adjusted the mattress, then he got a thinner pillow from his truck—patted it down and put it under his head and said, "See there, he is much lower now; the covering won't touch his nose at all—plenty of room there."

But I was eight years old and my eye level met the brow of the pine box. And my uncle's nose—like a little peak on a distant horizon—rose to a point just above the casket's rim.

1

Two preachers eulogized my uncle before the open casket at the church. They each preached a long time and kept pointing upward and assuring us that our dear departed was going to heaven. I felt good about what was being said, but I just couldn't keep my eyes off that little pinnacle on the casket's edge as I watched the flat top placed on the box and saw my relative's nose pressed down.

Later, in front of a mirror, I pushed my nose down with my fingers and said some words. The sound of my voice was strange. To say the least, I deemed it an awful thing to spend eternity with a flattened out nose and talking funny.

In the course of my next sixty years I have discovered much more about the life to come. To me heaven is a place where death does not exist—a city—not seen, but hovering eminently above us. Intuitively the whisper of faith ensures that our God and our deceased loved ones are alive and veritably closer than we can know. This good news should have a joyful impact on all persons.

Moreover, in God's celestial city there are no imperfections. My uncle left his compressed nose in the grave, and when I see him again he will be flawless. Above all, for you who are paradise bound, there is a bright and glorious future awaiting you in Abraham's bosom.

The apostle's words are right on target when he says, "Eye hath not seen, nor ear heard, neither have entered into the heart of man, the things which God hath prepared for them who love Him" (1 Corin. 2:9). Comfort each other with these words.

THE GIGGLES

It's possible that you—like me, are convinced that "giggling" is a form of human melody—an affliction that attacks certain persons suddenly, without warning, any place, any time.

My logic for this hypothetical reasoning is that I have never seen nor heard a fish, beast or fowl giggle. Also, by past standards, the concept that giggles are confined to young girls needs to be laid to rest. Fact is, no age or gender is immune to this condition. As for myself I've always been an inveterate giggler.

Seriously, now, has anyone ever thoughtfully attempted to define what a giggle is? I doubt it. That being the case let's explore the word and possibly uncover a few of its characteristics so that, perchance, some of its onslaught upon us may be curbed. Books of reference academically make an effort to describe the word as something like—repeated seizures of nervous laughter. Such analysis couldn't be further from the truth. Apparently, the authors of such wordings never had the giggles.

More to the point, a giggle is not a pleasant laugh, smile nor grin. Neither is it a robust laugh, simply because these expressions can be somewhat controlled mores of society. People can turn them on and off at will.

On the other hand, however, a giggle is a singular species in its own right. Unlike other pleasant demeanors it rarely can be controlled. If it is not allowed to come through the mouth on demand, it will explode via the nose, eyes and ears. Woe unto those with a mouthful of drink or food when a giggle attack comes.

For example, a sudden giggle blitz will grab the upper torso and rack it with tremors bringing forth the ungovernable utterances unattainable by normal laughter. And, too, giggles almost consistently strikes its victim at places best not to have them; especially in areas such as a worship service,

Sunday school, weddings, the dinner table, and when a brother is having a quiet talk with Dad to and from the woodshed.

In spite of all this, though, when I recall my giggle episodes I find the memories quite gratifying. In one sense I feel those hilarious eruptions of ungoverned mirth were good for my soul for most of mine occurred in God's house.

One lively happening in my young days was when my friend, Ted, got his right forefinger cut off just below the knuckle fooling around a carpenter shop. There was lamentation and stress all over town at little Teddy's misfortune.

But none of this kept him from Sunday church. My brothers and friends along with Teddy usually sat together in a certain section of the sanctuary. However, because of Teddy's accident he sat with his mother nursing his thumb and three and a half fingers in a bandanna sling. We boys, seated nearby, watched our little pal with sad sympathetic countenances—our tender heart mourning his loss.

By the third Sunday, however, the swelling in Teddy's hand had receded and his bandage loosened. Settled comfortably by his mother he was in full view of us boys. Quietly getting our attention he slipped the white dressing from his hand and wiggled his shortened finger vigorously at us.

We began to giggle. Then he put his nub in his nose and commenced twisting it ... stretching his lips downward. We all detonated and in a millisecond I saw Mama's austere facial features snap in our direction.

On top of that, I think the preacher thought we were laughing at him and he began dressing us down. Momentarily, we managed to restrain the giggling but Teddy wasn't through yet. He cocked his head to one side, put the remains of his finger in his ear and shook it intensely. By then our giggling was out of control. Mama jumped up, came back to where we were and marched us out.

For all practical purposes, retribution was at hand, but we still couldn't stop giggling. When we got home we told Mama what happened and she, too, began giggling. The contagion caught dad and he burst forth. Whew!

I was relieved—but we received stern warning—it was to never happen again.

I've heard a lot of sounds coming from the mouths of people in my day. All too many are agonizing words of troubles and distresses … very little humor.

In all truth, a happy heart laughs—even giggles. So parents if your children sometimes do some giggling—even in a worship service—don't get all that excited. They may have their eyes on a little Teddy sitting by his mother.

So give some thought to where you are. Truly, it is in the presence of God, and God loves a cheerful person. "A merry heart maketh a cheerful countenance" (Proverbs 15:3). So delight yourself in Christ Jesus and let Him smile on you and you be sure to smile back at Him.

I HATED RED HAIR

When in elementary school my hair was as red as a watermelon heart and I hated it. To make things worse—the only other carrot top in the whole school—from first grade to the twelfth—was a girl in my class.

At recess someone would inevitably suggest letting the two red-heads skip rope together. I didn't want to do that because I didn't like girls anymore than my crimson hair.

Under persistence, though, I usually gave in and hopped with my counter part to the gyrating rope while our peers chanted in cadence, "Red-headed woodpeckers, hopping on a pine—wants to chew tobacco—but can't have mine." Predictably, ardent giggles and mirth accompanied these indignities.

Obviously, I faced an ongoing dilemma out of control. What could I do to avoid these embarrassing occurrences in the future? We were oddities in the entire universe and appointed to suffer the abuse that went along with it.

But a problem will somehow get worked out. In time, a friend told me how to rid myself of my off-color nemesis. Of course, it would require some radical act on my part. So what? I was more than ready to do any thing to "change my leopard spots" (Jer. 13:23), and make me black haired like my friends.

With that sound advice, I followed my pal's formula to the letter. I made a concoction of melted Vick's Salve mixed with chimney soot and dyed the hair on my head, arms and eyebrows into a luxuriant, raven like finish.

That done, I looked at all of me in the mirror. Wow! I was breathtakingly handsome. I turned this way and that, admiring my deep dark hair and freckles. I smiled and my remodeled image grinned back—I liked what I saw.

My next step was to trot down town to my Dad's store and show the "new me" to my parents. Their response was swift. Back home we went, and after some vociferous compelling, amidst mountains of soap suds, kerosene and ungentle scrubbing I returned to my natural state.

Redheads, indeed, were few in number when I was a kid. No more. They have multiplied many times over. My younger brother—also a redhead—believed the cardinal tops will eventually take over the world. Teasingly, when he sees scarlet locks he intones with bold verification, "See, there goes another one of us."

Not surprising, practicing Christians are in the minority, like the redheads of long ago. So wouldn't it be healthful and healing for humankind if religious persons began to multiply and fill society with God's love and good works. Then when someone's kindness is observed we could remark, "See, there goes another one of us."

Don't be ashamed of the Spirit of God in you. And by all means don't hide it with worldly disguises such as Vick's Salve and smut. It's too hard to wash off.

TELEPHONES

There was time—not too long ago—when my generation lacked the modern high tech conveniences such as dial and touch-tone phones, nor trifles like cordless telephones with pull-out antennas, cellular phones and answering machines. Nevertheless, we had phones more sufficient for bona fide personable service than today's state-of-the-art fancies.

Most likely we would have rejected those ultra-modern, curvy, colorful gadgets and kept our plain old communication devices. You see, ours were solid—made to last, no-nonsense contraptions encased in sturdy rectangular boxes, stained brown and anchored to the wall in a suitable listening, talking place.

In the upper center of our stout phones—protruding like a miniature fog horn was the adjustable transmitter. And, cradled in the two-pronged holder on one side was the receiver. On the opposite perimeter was the hand crank to signal the switchboard operator that a call was coming in.

Fortunately, my town had its very own telephone office, managed by ... let's call her Mrs. Jones. Mrs. Jones connected all calls verbally and by hand. She was a forever resident and knew much about everyone and learned more about them every day. With delight, she exercised the defacto privilege to listen in on all telephone conversations ... often becoming the arbitrator in heated discussions, even to the point of solving family spats—or at least trying. Of course, if your call was confidential you politely informed Mrs. Jones not to listen—and she didn't, she said.

Clearly, our switchboard operator was a remarkable source of social benefits to her community. For instance, you might want to talk to so and so. Mrs. Jones recognized your voice immediately and called you by name, and might say, "Okay, I think he's home ... let's give it a try." Or she might tell you your party has gone to the doctor or is taking a nap—so call back after 4:00 p.m. She kept in touch with the sick, gave the time of day, what time church and Sunday School started and what was playing at the picture show. Indeed, if you wanted information or advice, call the telephone office.

Today, I call someone and get an answering machine. Other times I get a computer voice telling me my order is in. I dial a company about my account and a recorder directs me to press a number … another instructs me to punch more numbers. Then comes the extended waiting music. Eventually another tape admonishes me to not hang up—all lines are busy—the next available operator will take your call and on it goes. Oh, Lord, how I long to hear the voice of Mrs. Jones at yesterday's telephone office … so real—so affable—so unmechanical.

But the wind has passed all too quickly. Today becomes yesterday and tomorrow becomes today and the change is radical—time alters all things physical, including telephones. Yet there is one entity that time cannot recast. Our God does not transmute. "I am the Lord." He says. "I change not" (Malachi 3:6).

By gone times, however, provide lessons and blessings for us all. To reach the unchanging One, we do not have to press keys and listen to machine-driven voices. We dial our heavenly Father by simply calling His name and He promptly answers us. And, His grace is forever the same.

In a way, I like to compare Jesus with Mrs. Jones, the telephone operator. He is so real—so personable and so delighted to receive our calls. Why not give him a ring today?

THE TURKEY SECRET

Long before the emergence of Technicolor movies, an uncle of mine was a country doctor. He was, indeed, a compassionate fellow and felt such a deep humane responsibility for poor families that he would set them up in business raising turkeys on a share, share basis.

He, of course, would assume the expense of furnishing the turkey chicks along with feed—shelter and fence. When the turkeys were grown and sold, he, in turn, would receive half the proceeds.

One particular household who took him up on his offer was a man—his wife—a dirt yard full of barefoot children and an old, blind grandma who sat in a rocking chair by the fireplace puffing on a corn cob pipe day in and day out.

Eventually, when the turkeys should have grown enough to have commercial value, the doctor called upon the family to inspect the flock. But, alas, there were no fowl to survey and no money and no explanation to what had happened. Later, it was learned that the temptation was simply too great and the poor folks had eaten the birds.

Such behavior, understandable, didn't set too well with my uncle. In time he dropped in on the man to discuss the matter. They all sat around the fireplace—the husband, wife, barefoot children and blind grandma smoking her pipe.

"Tell me what happened to the turkeys," the doctor asked.

There was utter stillness for some overly long moments but my uncle probed further. "Did you sell them? Did someone steal them?"

For about five minutes the whole family said nothing, but looked sheepishly at the floor biting and pursing their lips. Grandma rocked, puffed, and blew smoke. The hush remained unbroken for several more minutes.

In effect, it had been quiet for so long that blind grandma assumed my uncle had left so she took the pipe our of her mouth and drawled, "Is he gone? Why didn't you just tell him the turkeys died with the sorehead? He wouldn't know the difference no way."

One might imagine the old lady's consternation when she suddenly realized the doctor was still there. Fortunately for them, though, the good physician had a forgiving heart—a sense of humor and continued to help this wondrously penitent family.

This story, in truth, has much to do with a little read Bible verse that warns, "curse not the King, no, not in thought; and curse not the rich man in thy bed chamber, for a bird of the air shall carry the voice, and that which hath wings shall tell the matter" (Eccl. 10:20). In other words—bad secrets are almost impossible to keep.

On a higher plane, however, no one can keep a secret from God "… his eyes behold, his eyelids try the children of men" (Ps. 11:43). And Jesus himself apprises all people that before God, "nothing is secret that shall not be shown; neither anything hidden, that shall not be known and come to light" (Luke 8:17).

This should be sobering information for all humankind under the realization that God knows everything. One day, the apostle admonishes, "God shall judge the secrets of men by Jesus Christ …" (Romans 2:16).

Confession is always good for the soul. So make known your secrets to God daily—remembering all can have an advocate with God in Jesus Christ the righteous who speaks for his subjects day and night. So keep Him working on your behalf and He will keep turkey secrets out of your closet.

YANKEE RUBBISH

Before the horse and buggy faded—altogether, from the South's Main Street—my brother and I saw a clerk stocking a shelf in our dad's store with odd shaped cans we had never seen the likes before.

They were red and modeled after miniature log huts with tiny chimney spouts. The label on each little house read, "Log Cabin Syrup," and in small print, "from New York State."

Curiosity, at once, fired my brain—and I unscrewed a wee lid from a chimney, but a covering of silver foil closed the opening. No problem, at all. I got a straight pin and when nobody was looking I pricked the thin seal and my brother and I took turns sucking a little of the succulent sapidity from the pygmy hut.

Wow! I never imbibed anything so sweet and delicious in all my life. The unfamiliar taste of sugary maple did, indeed, ravishly delight my palate, and I was—in mid moment, wholly addicted to something downright foreign and so … unconfederate.

And from my brother's rapt visage I knew he, too, had suddenly accrued and irresistible affinity for the candy juice from Lincoln's country.

Sometime later—after indulging every log cabin, we recapped the tops tightly and stacked them back in rows exactly as we found them. Furthermore, in the afterglow of our new found craving we gave our mother no rest until she put one of those log cottages from heaven's pantry on the breakfast table.

By contrast, however, that elfin hut of Yankee made nectar sitting alongside the tall pewter pitcher with the image of Robert E. Lee engraved on both sides and holding granddad's sugar cane syrup seemed all too revolutionary to say the least.

Our Mother's dad was not a large man, but he was, without exception—a giant in principle and conviction—mighty in faith and truly an ardent son of the south. We grandchildren loved him dearly and called him "Pa".

When Pa spoke of syrup he meant the sugar cane variety—thick and oozy—made form his own crop, grown on his farm. My brother and I happily accompanied him many times on cold autumn days when he hauled his stalks to the mill to have the juice crushed out and cooked into syrup.

Ice cold cane juice on those frosty mornings was nothing less than a beverage from Paradise. And Pa would happily intone, "Drink it down boys and tell me you like it." We did and he smiled upon us.

When the syrup was ready to be poured into buckets, Pa would strip off a piece of cane peeling—dip it into the syrup—taste it—smack his lips and say, "Boys, that's mighty good syrup—here, put some in your mouth."

We would take his peeling and do the same—smack our lips and say, "That sure is mighty good syrup, Pa." And Pa would grin—pat us on the head and say, "Now, that's my boys."

Against this backdrop, it was Pa's custom to pop in most any morning and eat breakfast with us. On this particular day it was biscuits, butter and syrup. With high visibility and without a care my brother and I deluged our buttered bread with Log Cabin Syrup form New York State and Pa inquired, "What's that mess you boys are pouring on your biscuits?"

"It's maple syrup from the store, Pa," my brother sang out. "We sure like maple syrup better than cane syrup now ... want to eat some with us?"

Intuitively, my natural proclivity told me that the most favored status my brother and I held with our grandpa had unexpectedly found itself treading on a sagging foundation. And by any account, my brother's innocent confessions didn't help one bit.

In the second, there fell upon our table an awesome stillness. It seemed the earth and all therein, had abruptly become silent and foreboding. Pa's face had turned to granite and Mama and Dad's eyes darted back and forth at each other.

It was quite obvious my brother and I had transgressed grievously and we squirmed under the nagging load of our exposed violation. To make matters worse our parents uttered no word of support on our behalf, and I called upon a higher power, "Lord, if thou wilt, have mercy on my brother and me."

Eons later, Pa's body finally stirred. He reached over and picked up the little maple house. He put on his glasses and read the label—then poured some in a spoon, like medicine—tasted it—smacked his lips—grimaced, and blurted, "Yuck! This isn't syrup—it's Yankee rubbish … too dark, too sweet and too thin. Colored sugar water is all it is. Here, read the label."

He leaned over and held out the alien shack to me. I cringed and scoured my brain for an appropriate appeasement acceptable to Pa. Then I just sputtered out, "Pa, we don't like this Yankee rubbish no more, no sir … we sure do like cane syrup now." And I reached for Robert E. Lee.

Pa leaned back in his chair—paused a moment—grinned and drawled, "Well, now, that's my boys."

After that, I forever deemed it an outright must to never, ever, eat maple syrup or any other foreign food in Pa's presence again. So we sopped biscuits in cane syrup and watched Pa beam with joy and cheerfully ring out, "Eat some more, boys, and tell me it's good."

But, alas, the delectable taste of sweet maple had already bonded with my southern taste buds, and ever now-and-then—when no one was watching, I pricked the foil on a tiny chimney spout, and savored again, the forbidden Yankee rubbish made for angels to drink.

Over my many years I've often thought of those syrup days and how they underscore why we are the way we are and our intense difficulty in accepting and tolerating unaccustomed things—unfamiliar people and their accents and ways.

The greater cause, of course, lies in the preconditioning of self begun in early childhood when the mind is indelible and attitudes and habits are easily formed. Fortunately, undesirable traits can be broken and bad attitudes can be altered—even down to syrup. But sometimes it must be forced.

For example, I was on the whole, at one time quite prejudiced and discriminatory. Yet it was not until I found myself in the midst of many individuals in the US Navy did I learn to appreciate fellas from different regions of the country—folks of different color, unfamiliar ways and peculiar enunciation's.

Some Yankee boys, oddly enough, soon became cherished friends of mine. In fact, I even got to liking northern food almost as much as my beloved southern victuals.

So how do you bring wrongful preconceptions to heal? From my standpoint the two most important approaches are, first, expose yourself to people not of your kind and their way of life with an open heart and mind.

Then reread the New Testament story of the Good Samaritan found in Luke 10:29-37, and you might surprisingly discover that the rejected half-breed Samaritan can represent every color and class on earth.

Strive to be kind and helpful like him and you will surely find the Lord is good and gracious and is apt to smile upon you—pat you on the head, and say, "That's my boy." It will be the smartest move you ever made.

THE SCHOOL LUNCH

Before the advent of automatic gear shifts in auto's, one of the most telling contrasts between town and country children took place at the school lunch hour. The hinterland schoolers brought their food—either wrapped in a paper or in a tin syrup bucket and ate on the playground. City kids went home to eat ... yours truly was a city kid.

Just observing my rural classmates happily dining on the grass suggested picnicking and I, indeed, loved picnics. Fact is, I was so eager to join them that I incessantly badgered my mother until she prepared a meal for me to take to school.

Exhilarated was I as she stacked an abundance of nutriments into a brown bag from dad's store. Wow, I could hardly wait for the dinner bell in class that day. But the time finally arrived and I joyfully sat down on God's good earth to break bread with my chum's from the countryside.

Then, amidst their unbroken chatter and laughter agrarian's offspring promptly began removing lunches from containers. A Strident buddy was excitedly telling us about the best coon hunt he had ever experienced.

Out of a paper wrap came an enormous biscuit—run through with a link of smokehouse sausage that jutted out about four inches from each side. A shiny pail produced a small mayonnaise jar full of black eyed peas mixed with cane syrup, and a pone of crackling corn bread on the side. In other hands appeared fried eggs, brown laced and sandwiched between two biscuit halves and some parched peanuts.

I, in turn, brought forth delicacies from my unwrinkled sack. Gently, I removed my mother's cloth napkin and spread it on the ground. On it I placed my light bread sandwiches ... all inlaid with mayonnaise, sliced bologna, boiled ham, pineapple slices and tuna salad.

Next came my wedge of Wisconsin State cheese, yellow as gold and wrapped in wax paper. I sat out my bottle of Nehi orange crush and began tearing the wrapper off my five cent box of saltine crackers.

Then, ready to join in the banquets, I looked up. The coon hunt had died on the wing. No one was chewing or swallowing—no one was talking, instead, all eyes were riveted on my snack from the town store.

Twenty minutes later we were finished and all I got from my lunch was a sip or two of orange crush. All the rest was traded for down-home cooking.

Now, some sixty years later I still recall that delightful happening because it had, for me, far reaching implications and provided me with many cherished memories. I doubt if any of my long ago classmates ever knew how much their lunches influenced my eating habits.

By all accounts, over the years, I have consumed large quantities of cold cuts, sandwiches and saltine crackers from the supermarket. But as good as those eats were they can never compare with the spicy savor of a country sausage distended about four inches from each end of a homemade biscuit.

Our Maker, unquestionably, has provided persons with many tasty things to eat, but for me, few dishes are as delectable as cane syrup poured on black eyed peas and eaten with crackling corn bread.

Clearly, there is a needful lesson in all this. For example, each personality is a unique banquet of good things to share with others that no one else has. It may be a talent—a knowledge, a laugh, an encouragement, a prayer, a comfort ... the list is endless.

All we have and are is a gift from God. They are his endowments to us and are not to hold, but to exchange. We are made that way. He has created us "fearfully and wonderfully" (Ps. 139:14) to be the spice of life to each other. Happy you will be if you do.

LITTLE CHICKENS

On my tenth birthday a dear old aunt ingeniously arranged to have a plump bantam hen with ten fresh hatched chicks to give me as a present. I was, indeed, happily ecstatic over her thoughtful gift and eagerly looked forward—after that ... to my lucky day each year.

In the meantime, I nurtured my colorful feathered largess and her off-spring with enthusiastic care. However, as time passed I soon discovered that bantam poultry—like sparrows—mature quickly and multiply even faster.

Then, too, another year hurriedly rolled around and new batches of cheeping balls of down had swelled my growing flock considerably. In short, my ever increasing cock-a-doodle-doo's and clucking assets began to weigh heavy upon me, and Dad warned unsympathetically, "too many, son."

Bantam chickens, or bannies, as we called them, are about half the size (maybe less) of ordinary domestic fowl. But what they lack in body weight is made up in sheer beauty, courage and smart-alecky cockiness ... but lovely to look at and easy to adore.

As rounded and cute, though, as the small hens were, they never wore the colorful plumage of their male counterpart. But their lovely feathers of somber shades and hues beheld an aesthetics all their own.

By contrast, the roosters' attire was, in fact, pronounced and spectacu-lar. Their rainment bore brilliant streaks, blotches and sweeps of purple, green, chestnut, reds, orange, ad infinitum ... as if they had just hopped out of a festive, oriental painting.

But despite their marked handsomeness and diminutive stature they—by nature—were conceited, egotistical, feisty show-off's, and believed their crow to be mightier than the great Rhode Island Red King. These miniature upity-ups did not walk, and scratch and peck like common fowl … they strutted and pranced, tapped and nibbled as though they were the arbiters of chicken table manners and social behavior.

And, so, my little chickens proliferated like the Hebrews in Egypt until I owned eighty-eight of the stunted darlings. They crowed and clucked—laid tiny eggs and paraded and flaunted themselves. Their radiant feathers flashed everywhere—in the garden, trees, the yard, road and front and back porches. They were lovely, happy birds and I wanted hundreds, but Dad's notice wasn't to be taken lightly. On top of that I overheard him tell Mama, "Those bannies are ruining the garden."

Realizing my gorgeous dears were becoming a nuisance, I worried at what Dad might do if they continued making a chicken yard out of his garden. Mind you, I had seen him bring down many quail with his twelve gauge, and my insides got queasy when I imaged the air over his vegetable plot filled with zillions of tiny, wafting feathers and little croaking bodies on the ground.

Befuddled and anxious, I attempted every means to keep my petite gems out of Dad's rows of plants. Clipping their wing tips to prevent them from flying over the fence didn't work. They simply squeezed through the narrow wire meshes.

Making mock snakes out of hoses and old belts and laying them, along with an aged coonskin on the soil had no affect either. They frolicked and feasted right beside their imitation predators. Every endeavor to shoo them from Dad's domain failed. For their own welfare I finally put the word out, "Bannies for sale."

It was then a country friend came to my rescue and told me he would swap thirty-five pigeons for my eighty-eight plus bannies. Since pigeons were not garden molesters Dad agreed whole heartedly. So, in short order, a band of cooing birds replaced my bannies, and I promptly loved them as much.

My brother helped me build a wire cage for my birds, but it wasn't large enough for flying fowl. Dad suggested turning them loose—and I suspect—hoping they would fly away forever. In case they did, I tearfully said goodbye to my pigeons and set them free. But to my rapt delight, they only moved to the kitchen roof where the overhang of the higher shingles gave them shelter.

Like my bannie adventure I quickly learned that pigeons were more fruitful than chickens and I, before long, possessed a numberless flock living over the kitchen and even extending above Mama's bedroom. My mother couldn't stand the bird's mournful cooing at night ... said it sounded like ghosts.

But, they continued to proliferate and I was elated and loved the night sounds they made. I still had them when I left for the navy in WWII, but when I returned they were gone. I sort of let it go at that and made no inquiries.

From those growing up years, though somewhat problematic at the time, I later discerned that such happenings as this demonstrated what God had in mind when he said he would "open you the windows of Heaven and pour you out a blessing that there shall not be room enough to receive it" (Malachi 3:10B).

But, for me, those heightened material assets didn't shine as bright while watching my saintly aunt walking down the hill to our home ... bearing in a small box of straw a gift of one bantam hen and ten peeping chicks.

Her sweetness sparkled as a clear day when she gave her birthday boy his prize. Of course, the precious contents of her container were exuberantly accepted and cared for and grew until the excess was simply too much.

My aunt was a cheerful giver and her smile was that of an angel. By all accounts God loves those who imparts to others ungrudgingly, and especially does He relish the sound of angel laughter coming from humans, because He, Himself, is a joyful provider, and He desires His people to be like Him and have full joy.

Such is a lesson to practice. It returns remarkable dividends and underscores that paramount truth, "give and it shall be given unto you; good measure, pressed down, and shaken together, and running over ..."(Luke 6:38). My aunt was a living testimony to that truth.

So, why not give it a try? Smile—laugh—be a cheerful giver, learn of your Creator and see if He doesn't smile and laugh along with you and shower you with an overflow of the abundant life and well being.

PETER BLUE

When we were young, my brother and I bought ourselves barlow jack-knives for ten cents each. We were so excited over our new pocket cutlery we just couldn't wait to show them to our dad for approval ... even though we knew better.

Dad's response, as he examined our treasured cutting tools was, "hmmm." He opened the blades—touched their sharp tips and again said, "hmmm." Then he pushed the blade points into a crack in the floor and broke them off. That, said he, was to keep us from sticking ourselves when we fell off the fence. Henceforth, we were called the "no point" brothers.

The creepy old man who presided over the city pound was said to be half Indian. He wore old overalls, three sizes too large, and a dusty black hat that shaded two wide open eyes. His grin showed three long teeth. A deep pocket, corn sack hung on one shoulder and a nine foot leather whip coiled around the other.

He could be seen near the end of the day on the dirt road—dropping some grains of corn and a little food now and then while some hogs—a cow or two—maybe a few goats, followed the bait to the animal jail.

When the animals became disorderly he need only take the whip's handle and the thing seemed to come alive and uncoil by itself. A slight movement of the arm—a flick of the wrist—a loud crack, and immediate obedience swept over the arrested stock.

People called him Crow, but we town boys knew his real name was Peter Blue. Blue, so we had heard, caught bad kids and took them off in his sack and beat them up good with his whip or just killed them outright.

Furthermore, he could—at night, even change himself into a solid black wildcat. That was certainly so because his eerie caterwauling could be heard out there in the dark causing young skins to chill and crawl.

"There ain't no such thing as Peter Blue, is there?" I anxiously asked my uncle in the small hours after hearing a long catty bawl from under the house.

"Well, son, let's hope not," was his ominous answer. Indeed, definitely nothing reassuring there.

The six blocks from the movie house to where we lived had no night time street lights. There were only the great foreboding oaks casting sinister shadows over the path homeward—and a still scarier Baptist church with its huge white double doors ... also shrouded in fearful shadowy patterns.

When my brother and I went to the picture show, our sister, most of the time, had to come along with orders from Dad, "You boys look after your sister." No argument there, we knew to do exactly that.

In that environment we three saw, one evening a horrific Werewolf movie, and Werewolf shows always produced darker nights than usual.

After the show our little legs hurried us homeward in an anxious trot. Our sister was between us as we neared the church.

As we were passing the Lord's house those great white double doors—for no known reason—screeched wide open. Instantly, my brother gasped, "Peter Blue," And like tiny mosquitoes caught in a rush of wind my brother and I vanished. A half block away—pell mell in flight, the realization hit us that our sister wasn't with us.

Looking back I saw her standing like a pillar of salt in front of those gaping doors and I recalled Dad's firm directive, "You boys look after your sister." In a wink our pointless blades were in our hands. Back we flew ... grabbed a hand each and raced for home.

On the front porch, with sister safe inside and Dad close by my brother and I courageously traversed our verandah as undaunted as little dogs bravely barking in the safety of a fenced yard. Stridently, we invited man or monster to show himself. We waved our blades and made stabbing gestures in the dark as we hurled threatening expletives into the night. Whatever was out there better wise up and realize who they were dealing with ... or else.

All at once, in the midst of our fearless tirade there erupted—from under the porch, a low moaning yowl. It could mean only one thing: Peter Blue. Instantly, our knives fell to the floor and the no point brothers, terrified, frantically sought to enter the door at the same time crying out hysterically, "Dad! Dad! Help! Peter Blue, Peter Blue!"

In the house, Dad, awakened, and obviously weary of hearing Peter Blue and bawling cat stories set his two fright-shocked boys down at the kitchen table. After calming our fears he sternly scolded us for allowing our common sense to turn dumb.

He had known old Crow for years, he said. And he does the community an outstanding service—working long hours keeping the streets free of loose live stock. By all means we should appreciate his labor and be ashamed to think he would harm anyone. And another thing, the only mischief howling cats can do is keep people awake at night.

Oddly enough, Dad had one warm commendation for us. I told you boys, said he, to look after your sister. In that you did good and you showed considerable courage in doing so. You did your duty and I'm proud of you both.

Well, as the years passed by, Dad, eventually let us keep the points on our knives, but it took us a little longer to water down our bugaboo of Peter Blue and meowing cats on those dark nights.

The word duty, though, has been a part of me since Dad brought it to my attention at the kitchen table long ago.

Most significant, however, was my discovery that duty is a paramount importance in a person's life function. It also has much to do with one's relationship with God. "Fear God, and keep his commandments: For this is the whole duty of man," reads the ancient Oracle (Eccl. 12:13B).

Doing your duty is genuinely essential to your faith walk and character. Without it, two important keys to the good life, conviction and personality, are fundamentally compromised and one may find himself shut off from intended blessings.

The point is that duty to God and neighbor must take priority over feelings. Duty, too, is doing the right thing regardless of opposition and necessity.

For example, I may not feel loving today, but duty demands I show compassion. I may be angry and inclined to speak harshly but duty commands me to talk softly. Suppose my generosity is at a low ebb, nevertheless my charge is to be benevolent. Doing duty, by and large, keeps us aware of our daily up and down sensibilities.

Great rewards are prepared for those who do their duty toward God and man. So make every effort to do what the Lord of heaven and earth require; or, you too, on some dark night, just might encounter Peter Blue with a pinched off barlow blade to prove your worth.

MAMA HAD TOE POWER

In my family the two major modes of discipline that kept us children in line was voice power and toe power. Both held equal, authoritative license. Dad need only call the child's name once—and he knew to do his bidding.

Mama, on the other hand, took an unorthodox, but effectual, route to maintain order among her chicks. As quickly as a fly she could reach out with her foot—grab some leg calf between her big toe and the adjacent one—do a half twist, and her subject was suddenly stricken with pain and motion loss. No question there, Mama had toe power ... unlimited—even proficient enough to pinch through her stocking feet.

Not to be left out, though, I, too, had inherited some toe craft, albeit, on a more benign but noisy level. I could—at any time, make my right, big toe crack like a rifle or pistol when I bent it a certain way. I could cock, rapid fire or single shot, what ever the occasion required and never misfire.

The rule at bedtime, traditionally, was for us kids to be quiet and go to sleep. But my toe play was nocturnal and at its best in the night. Unfortunately, my late hour recreation ran smack into Dad's slumber agenda.

Our home was made of pine boards, resting high above the ground on brick pillars. The north wind in winter flowed at will beneath the woodwork chilling the floor to near freezing—keeping the house air shivery, but the beds were cozy and warm.

We were five brothers and one sister. Four boys slept in the back room on two big double beds. Sis had a room all to herself. The baby sibling slept at the foot of mama's bed in cold weather. But Mama couldn't tolerate anything crowding her feet. So when her wee lad got too close she tendered a mild toe tweak sending the little fella yipping and scurrying back to his allotted spot.

My toe frolicking—quite obviously, was next to impossible to manage. After the lights were turned out I would lie in bed and relive a western movie I had seen. In fantasy I eagerly joined the cowboys in shoot-outs. My toe gift leaped into action and emulated the bang, bang reports of gunfire which, of course, was the only sound heard in the dark.

Dad, in the next room would call my name only one time. Without delay I knew to cease fire—blow the smoke from my gun barrel and flip it into its holster. But in a little while I forgot and started shooting all over again.

The next happening was hearing the bed springs squeaking as Dad got up—fumble for his paddle at the side of the wood box and feel its sting in the appropriate place. One swat the first time ... do it again, two swats, and so on. In desperation I finally learned to mute my wild toe with splint and wrapped with much toilet paper at bedtime.

Not surprising, my good ole dad could never understand Cowboy and Indian wars or cattle rustling. Neither could he fathom the delicate art of fanning the hammer on my make believe six shooter or working my Winchester 73 lever action rifle and blasting away using my toe for sound effect. As I rattled on his eyes seemed to fix on something out there, and I knew it was a nay.

But my toe proficiency paled beside my mother's. She had real toe power. A case in point was the time Dad was in the hospital in a distant city, and a wealthy uncle came to pay him a call. I drove Mama and this well-to-do relative to the medical center.

After the visit we went to a restaurant for lunch. When we finished the waitress placed the bill on the table. As I reached for it Mama bumped my leg to stop with her foot. I frowned my displeasure at her and almost had the ticket when she slipped her shoe off—shoved her toes against my leg—vised in skin and flesh and turned.

I was in lock-jaw pain. The motor part of my body froze—halting limb movement cold. My tongue lay flat and comatose as my arm remained extended, reaching for the tab. And Mama smiled and didn't let go until my uncle picked up the check and laid the tip on the table. Then she just beamed and chatted pleasantries to my kin as we left the cafe ... I with a slight limp.

Archaic as it may seem my parents knew the value of the Proverbs "to train up a child in the way it should go and, when he is old, he will not depart from it" (Prov. 22:6). One might be surprised how effective this formula is if carried out … even if it takes some toe action.

Mom and Dad realized, also, that for this ancient precept to succeed, the children must first be taught simple obedience: Not obedience that provokes, but a trained subjection that promotes respect for parent, fellow siblings, peers and neighbor—and that right early.

They, for certain, believed the spin-off of proper discipline was responsibility, reverence, honesty, courtesy, security and a host of other good character building attributes the offspring would certainly need to function suitably in society.

The question for my parents was: Did their method work?

Well, my sister and my brothers and I taught our children as our progenitors instructed us—except for Mama's hair-trigger toes. Now, some three score years later we still rise up and call Mama and Dad blessed and thank God for the way they raised us. Of corresponding importance our children and grandchildren have made us proud and we are again grateful to our Creator that we could pass it on to them.

So listen up, Mother and Father. If you've tried many modern techniques that haven't panned out, why not give old Proverbs 22:6 a try. Begin by teaching the kids basic obedience, and soon, or God just might reach down one day with his toes and give you a painful half-turn to remind you of its relevance.

IF YOU WERE THE DOG

A few houses up the street—in my neighborhood—lived a gorgeous, full grown collie dog. So handsome was this magnificent creature that I eyed him with ardent infatuation any time he sauntered by.

His coat and great mane was a luxuriant, fluffy tan and white. His eloquent stride was, indeed a moving portrait of grace and grandness. Even neutral and non-dog lovers noted that this animal's carriage and behavior disclosed an uncommon unity of natural sophistication and intelligence.

Favored superbly above his fellows with such prominent attributes the imposing dog did, unarguably, have it all together. And since he was so resplendent in all his endowments, my brothers and I—down the street—dubbed him "King".

But, in spite of King's notable record of excellence, he harbored one tiny blot on his otherwise reputable demeanor, and that was to prove his undoing. He loved to chase cats.

The lady across the street from us—with the orangy hair—was owned by an adorable, blue-gray Persian cat. The pretty feline's long silky fur was kept shiny clean, combed and downy puffed at all times. A pink ribbon bow perched beside her little kitty ear.

By any measure, the woman pampered the cat excessively and called her "my darling Princess." And the wise little princess purred and whined itsy-bitsy meows as her loving foster mother held her in her arms and cooed baby talk to her.

But then, there was another pitch to the voice of the cat's doting benefactor. When aroused it could burst forth into a shrill, grating screech capable of stopping cold, both man and beast, and rip asunder their nerve systems and bone marrow at the same time.

By and large, the darling kitty's range was confined to the safety of home and yard … except for that one day. Curiosity finally overtook Princess and she decided to slip away from her protective habitat for a while and explore the mysteries of her neighborhood. Unbeknownst to her, though, the bold enterprise would take her into the king's territorial domain.

There was a menacing snarl and the startled cat suddenly realized she desperately needed the security of her palace. So without even a passing hello she made the harrowing dash across no-cat's-land with the growling collie two perilous feet behind in hot pursuit.

My brothers and I across the road—on the front porch—began to take notice. The woman, seeing her darling's immediate danger rushed to the edge of her verandah—her tangerine hair ablaze—and hurled a fusillade of shrieks and screams at the dog I'm sure he had never heard before. The sound of a fast breaking freight train could not have matched the verbal onslaught. Momentarily, nature was shut down.

The scalding eruption threw up an invisible rock shield and caught the unsuspecting dog face on just as the cat leaped safely into the bosom of her mistress. The verbal bulwark brought the collie to a sudden, abrupt hault, and there he stood, motionless, seemingly suspended an inch or two above ground level.

In full view, a prodigious transformation crept over the splendid canine. His flashy mane and radiant coat turned pallid as one possessed. Whatever poise and finesse he held in his graceful body fled him now, unabated.

Defeated, the disheveled dog slowly turned homeward, and with tail between his legs he sort of tiptoed back to his kingdom, a stunned and altered monarch.

My brother correctly prophesized, "That dog is ruined—he'll never be fit for anything again." An occasional observation after that bore those facts out. Sad to say, a short time later his majesty developed a list to the right as he walked. His noble stride was gone. He never chased a cat again. A little petting would stimulate a feeble tail wag or two, but other than that the dog kept to himself.

And here I confess. I just couldn't resist embellishing this tale a little. However, my point is: if you were the dog, what was your character flaw that led to your misfortune? Chasing cats, of course, but to put it in perspective you could have avoided it all if you had been circumspect.

Scripture affords much credence to the word, circumspect. "See that ye walk circumspectly," advises St. Paul, "not as fools, but as wise" (Eph. 5:15).

Without doubt, this verse provides an excellent family and social rule for mannerly behavior. The axiom seriously coaxes persons to practice prudence when dealing with people. It counsels one not to act, speak, growl or bark discordantly toward others. By all means, take time to give thought to what you're about, and remember always, "a soft answer turneth away wrath: but grievous words stir up anger" (Pr. 15:1).

Circumspection calls for discreteness and sensitivity—considering all consequences. For instance, will someone be offended or hurt by what I do or say? In the encounter, will my relationship with my fellow woman and man be enhanced or diminished? Or, after the fact, will I be perceived as a disagreeable prig? All in all, will people want to avoid me?

There are some great benefits to prudent practice. It develops within you a discerning spirit that provides you peace, graciousness, health and a happy family and social life, to name a few.

So do what your maker intended for you all along. Conduct yourself properly among other humans. Or, like King, you might find yourself suspended in midair someday, crushed and dejected, and perhaps walking alone with a list to the right—or left—or both.

THE TONSIL FUNERAL

High school football and basketball coaches in the 1930's and early forties were happily delighted when prospective athletes had their tonsils removed. They believed, along with most parents, that the kid—after those bad organs were cut out—would devour colossal amounts of food and drink, and by Fall be a foot taller and twenty pounds heavier—needed bulk for the team.

My formative years were cast in those almost pre-antibiotic times. Against this backdrop, it seemed all my pals, including myself—ached severely from tonsillitis during the flu season along with its swollen neck and sore throat.

Commonly prescribed medication for the affliction was usually two or three drops of kerosene or turpentine in a spoon of sugar each day with thorough applications of Vick's salve rubbed into the skin and meat of the neck and chest. Characteristically, though, this regimen only produced the sinking feeling of burial preparations for the victim and did little to heal the sickness.

However, there was a second option if the first medicament was unsuccessful. That, of course, was to have the inflamed lymphoid surgically extracted. Indeed, this prognosis, if pursued, would do the job—put color in the face, and add weight and energy to the body's composition. Everybody knew that coaches waxed ecstatic when they heard an athletic youth was having a tonsillectomy.

My parents chose the tonsil operation for me and I was propitiously elated because the value of its fringe benefits far out weighed any thoughts of pain. After all, I, too, like my puny peers with infected glands—aspired to be a star athlete—bowling over the opposition, making touchdowns and never missing a lay-up. But I weighed only ninety pounds … a lot of bark on skinny legs.

But in due course, at age thirteen—my tonsils were expurgated. I awoke from the anesthetic with an awful sore throat—but that was okay—I was going to fill out—grow taller—and play ball in the Fall.

Consolingly, my parents, sister and brothers stood by my bed speaking comforting words to me. Then when I was fully awake the doctor came in and told us he had a present for me and handed me a small glass vial containing my tonsils submerged in a clear holding fluid. Mama and my sister turned pale—grimaced and emitted together, "Euggh!" But wow! My brothers and I had never seen tonsils before. By any measure, we were simply fascinated with that little jar holding some stuff from inside you.

But if I could have read my mother's thoughts, I would have known the days of my small gift was numbered. At home she wouldn't let me keep them on the mantel above the fireplace—or on the dresser—or the kitchen table. And my sister went hysterical every time I tried to hand them to her. My small treasure had to stay in my room—out of sight—no exceptions, my mother warned. What's more, daily pressure was constantly upon me to dispose of my precious gift—and soon—like yesterday. They were disgustingly, sickening, my mother said.

Quite frankly, the die was cast, and after some painful deliberations—my brothers and I decided to have a funeral for my tonsils. That would obviously end the abuse I was sorely enduring. Sadly, we dug a little hole, placed the vial holding the dead bodies of my tonsils and made an oval shaped mound of earth over it, and placed a small cross at the head. We covered the tiny grave with some violets—sang a hymn and stood reverently as I said a prayer for them, "as I lay me down to sleep …" A brother wrote the epithet on a piece of paper and attached it to the cross "Here lies some of Joseph's bad innards, may they rest in peace." Mama and my sister breathed a sigh of relief.

But the news spread abroad and some cousins came with complex curiosity to see my tonsils. Simply put, there was nothing to do but exhume those wee corpses. So, they were back in the house again—but immediately out again—another funeral—another resurrection as friends and kin came and went.

Then one day I dug into the earth preparing for a viewing but my tonsils weren't there. I poked and scooped but my celebrities could not be found. I searched everywhere but discovered no remains. I never saw them again, but I suspected mama and my sister knew their whereabouts. Anyway, I guess it was for the best.

Unlike my ancient tonsil interments, many, to their good fortune, follow the apostle's advice and bury their old sin-loving nature and leave it there. But most—like me and my baneful tonsils—simply can't let the negatives stay in the grave. We call them forth—give them nourishment—give them the kiss of acceptance and place them in our hearts again.

Our souls, in reality, hold grudges, envies, hates, guilt and ultimately depressions. The list is endless of things that restrict the cognition and robs us of the good life. What can we do? This, in Christ God gives power to bury inner antagonisms and strength to ignore them.

And if, perchance, you, in time, inadvertently uncover your decomposed temptations, you might discover that God—like my mother and sister, has quietly removed them as far as the East is from the West and they trouble you no more. Give it a try.

CAN YOU SPELL CZECHOSLOVAKIA?

When it became quite evident the United States would soon enter World War II—President Roosevelt, in 1940, proposed with all expedience, that all male high school students take as much math as possible.

Presumably, to fight a war—boys must be able to move beyond the recitation of multiplication tables and the complexities of long division. Modern warriors must, in fact, learn to grasp, to some degree, the precision and intricate details of such enigmatic configurations as algebra—physics—geometry, trigonometry and calculus.

Across the nation, education departments and county school boards expeditiously took our commander-in-chief's mandate as a statute to be adhered to the letter.

As for me, though, I was intensely disappointed at that concept because there existed in my brain no propensity for equations, angles—triangles and symbols of little letters attached to digits.

Already I had read all of Jack London's books and decided to be a writer like him and not a mathematician. But the president's directive was no respect of person, and I soon found myself plunged unwilling into an unfamiliar arena of high mathematics.

Some of my friends, however, took off like Archimedes. To say the least, I was simply astonished at how they could brightly comprehend every computation written on the blackboard and understand with decoding alacrity the teacher's disparate works, and I couldn't.

I was filled with envy. Nevertheless, I taxed my brain striving to understand the imposing art of numbers because ultimately Germans and Japanese had to be whipped and math would do it. And I, for sure, didn't want to appear lacking in zeal for God and country. But my aptitude for math didn't improve and I began avoiding my ingenious classmates for embarrassment's sake. They spoke the Euclid jargon with relative ease and I, when there was no escape, smiled and nodded, pretending I understood precisely what was said. So it stands to reason why my self-esteem hovered near rock bottom.

Then, one day—a modicum of Serpentine wisdom wormed its way into my conscious. I knew some of those math whizzes couldn't spell any better than I ... some worse. Against this backdrop, I began to devise a plan to recover my lost self-approval among my colleagues and get back at them for knowing more than me. I learned to spell "Czechoslovakia."

And so, as we gathered in the hall or at the school concession bar some of the elite would discuss, adroitly, some sticky points in a matter-of-fact problem. It was on such an occasion that I interrupted and casually inquired, "Hey, did you guys know that there is a simple little word—with clear, distinct syllables—that a lot of students are having trouble spelling ... none of you, of course, but, well, it just seems strange to me?"

"What's the word?"

"It's Czechoslovakia, anyone of you could spell it, I'm sure ..."

Well, a couple of my Einstein pals took a shot at it and flunked the test. Then they exchanged glances and seemed unhappy that I had brought to bear upon them a less known subject.

"Let's hear you spell it," someone quipped.

"Okay," I said, as a surge of pure delight swept through me.

"C-Z-E-C-H-O-S-L-O-V-A-K-I-A!"

Sometime later I cast upon their natural inclinations for symbols and brackets a name for a common medicine to spell. "Asafetida." It produced the same results. Wow, I felt myself an equal, and my ego soared into the firmament.

I disclosed this experience because it stems from Jesus' advice to His Apostles, "be ye, therefore, wise as serpents, and harmless as doves" (Matthew 10:16B). Frankly, I erroneously thought I should be gentle among my peers, but also crafty like a snake—for when it becomes necessary the serpent knows when to strike back.

But Jesus did not mean it that way. Be wary, He would say, but not cunning. Develop a Christian instinct that avoids danger and temptations, like a serpent. And like a dove know your limitations and your strengths. Let false pride and envy be restrained and harmless. And by all means, may the wisdom and gentle love of the Master make you humble, wise and good.

Eventually, I learned some math.

THE DELIVERY TRUCK

I was large for my age at thirteen and my Dad owned a country store. He also had a delivery truck which I was happily learning to drive. It was also nineteen forty and the military draft had taken away so many young fellas that Dad could not find anyone to work at the store.

Actually, I was delightfully gratified to see those guys leave because their absence propelled me—unchallenged—into the driver's seat of the store truck. Consequently, there was no option for Dad but to allow me to haul feed, seed, fertilizer and groceries in the pickup. Ecstatic joy, indeed ran through my bones as I thought of shifting those gears—skidding those tires and honking the horn at my friends. Wow!

Since domestic telephones were scarce in those days I was on the store bicycle at daybreak going from house to house—ten miles a day—taking grocery orders. And since most homes in our town had chickens and cows I took feed orders as well.

After the purchases were filled at the store I then delivered them on the truck. I also was expected to haul tons of hundred-pound sacks of feed for mules and oxen to logging camps—a task I had not duly contemplated. But all this went along with truck driving privileges. It didn't take long, however, for me to get gruesomely weary of all this work.

But when there's a need, a way is provided to meet the wish, and this is where my friend, Curtis, steps into the picture. Curtis, indeed, was willing to give me—at least—half his kingdom if I would teach him to drive the truck.

So, on occasion I let him sit close to me and steer and shift gears until he actually learned to drive.

Suddenly, a glorious bright light flashed and I discovered a way to ease my burden of labor and catch up on my comic book reading at the same time.

To make that happen I presented a proposition to my friend he couldn't resist. If he would unload the groceries and feed at the proper places I would, in turn, let him do all the driving. Curtis took the bait and for many weeks I simply went along for the ride and read my comic books. Gee whiz, what a good life ... that is, until the awful day that ended it all.

My happy chauffeur's older sister operated a beauty shop in their family home and used vinegar by the gallon for hair rinses. It was a busy morning for her that day. She had a lady in every chair and was rapidly running out of vinegar. Curtis was dispatched to Dad's store to get six gallons of the stuff to be delivered immediately.

As for me, my friend couldn't have arrived at a better time. The truck was already filled with grocery and feed orders—ready to take out. I had also traded twelve comic books for a dozen I hadn't read and couldn't wait to get to them. Simply put, the sight of Curtis filled my soul with sheer gladness.

Convincingly, I told my friend if we hurried he could drive the truck—take the groceries in—and still get the vinegar to his sister in plenty of time ... at least I thought we could. But we were a mite late—about an hour or so. After all, what did I know about women in the beauty shop waiting for vinegar.

Curtis was a cheerful whistler, and upon arrival at his home—our last stop—he bounded through the front door, his lips melodiously pursed in birdsong. Then, abruptly, the whistling stopped. The next sound I heard was Curtis crying out to his mother, "Mama! Don't! Ouch! Mama ... My sunburn—O'Ouch!" Then I heard his mother shout in awesome focused anger, "Now where is that delivery boy?"

I, indeed, with all prudent foresight rapidly double-clutched my legs into passing gear—slid the case of vinegar onto the back porch and raced with all my might back to the truck. I knew then that the curtain to my delightful arrangement with Curtis was rapidly falling.

Not surprisingly, my pal's sister could wait no longer so she called the store. Dad sent the vinegar to her in a taxi.

I sat on a box in the back of the store, cringing under Dad's austere interrogation confessing all. After that, through expediency and much anxiety I gave avid attention to my delivery tasks for many days afterward.

Later in life I pondered how easy it is to succumb to charming enticements. People make choices. I chose to shirk my duties and became a tempter to Curtis and devised an arrangement he couldn't resist for my own benefit. This boyhood experience—as harmless as it was, nevertheless, underscores the power of human desire.

Many persons are obsessed with wants and superfluous cravings most of the time and will often do what is necessary to attain them—right or wrong. The attraction is, "I want what I want, now." Fact is, though, the consequences are hardly ever factored in, and they may be dire.

So, how does a person deal with wrong temptations? First, help is needed from heaven. Doesn't the Lord's prayer explicitly call upon the Creator to "Lead us not into temptation and away from evil." Recite it often. "Second, doesn't the Epistle declare that offensive allurements are a common happening to all humans, but a way out is always provided" (1 Cor. 10:13). Albeit, few find it, but they can.

Historically and Biblically God has made persons "fearfully and wonderful"

(Ps. 139:14). And has created them with the mental and physical capacity to strive against overwhelming odds and overcome them all. Indeed, this reality is little known, but should be etched in the heart and mind.

Furthermore, make the effort—learn how to exercise your God given power to resist unsound enticements. You can do it. If not, you too may find yourself on the vinegar run, or worse.

A COW TO MILK

In the home habitat of my juvenility there was certain indigenous tasks assigned my brother and me by our Dad. We got the firewood in—took care of the garden—cut the grass with a sling (no power mowers in those days), raked up the dead pine needles in the cow pasture—fed the chickens and slopped the hogs. Counterwise, our spoiled sister's work allocation was to milk the cow, and that was all she did.

Just watching her milk, though, simply fascinated me. Riveting, indeed, would be an appropriate assessment of my feelings as I observed her sitting on the stool—milk pail between her knees—both hands rhythmically pulling and squeezing and listening to the thin streams in perfect cadence hiss-hissing into the rising foam.

Simply put, I had to have that job for myself, and if I could swing it with Dad I thought, not only would I enjoy a super terrific chore, but, like my sister—I would be excused from all those uninteresting mundane work burdens my brother and I were stuck with.

Under the circumstances, however, persuading Dad to allow me to milk would be a daunting endeavor to say the least. As I expected, Dad was straightforward and to the point. "Nothing doing," he said, "it's you sister's job."

But, as always, rejection simply intensified my persistence. And so, my sister was my text target. I knew if I could persuade her to stop milking I was next in line. In this context I wheedled, cajoled and pleaded with her to tell Dad she didn't want to milk anymore. "Nope, I like to milk," was her reply. "I love my cow." I told her I loved the cow also and would give her my five ceramic elephants in Mama's china closet if she let me milk. "No."

In effect, nothing worked. But not to give up. Undeterred, I moved to plan two—force. Daily, by stealth and ambush, I strove to separate, for good, my sister from her milk pail. But, I soon discovered how deadly accurate she was at spurting the cow's milk long distance. She could drown a fly on the barn gate fifteen feet away. Fact was, every time I got near her I caught a stream of warm milk either in my ear, nose, mouth, eye, hair or clothes. But by George, I was going to milk that cow and nothing this side of eternity would stop me.

Thankfully, every good and fair boy has his day, and mine finally came one morning after a heavy rain that made mush out of the dirt, stall floor. At last, I succeeded in creeping up behind my sister as she milked. Gamely, I caught her by the hair of her head and yanked her off the stool into the barnyard soup. She screamed and cried and when I let go she ran to the house wailing hysterically, and I felt an uneasy sense of gratification. "Let her squall," I thought. "So what … shoot she didn't own the cow any-way—much mine as hers."

But an ill wind was blowing hard that day. Dad was home. And when I was apprised of that fact a still small voice spoke to my soul, "today you die." And the thought of the after math of my crime began to weigh heavy on my heart.

However, to my portentous surprise, Dad did not even lift the strap or raise his voice as I anticipated. Simply and calmly he spoke to me, "Son, from now on milking the cow is your cookie. No matter what, you will milk her every day—twice a day, along with all your chores."

Needless to mention, I was so delighted that my life had been spared that I failed to digest the ramifications of my new appointment, but hap-pily absorbed the sweet reality that all my efforts had paid off. Glory! I would live and milk the cow also. From now on the sweet old cow was mine. Oh, what a thrill it was for the next few days as I gleefully sang and whistled as I milked.

But then as the cycle of seed time—harvest time—cold, heat, summer and winter rolled over me, I was milking the cow every day, twice a day—year in—year out. Everywhere, anywhere I happened to be, I had to keep in mind to be home at milking time. My burden waxed great, and I developed an inordinate dislike for that dumb cow, her chalky milk, that pail and that stupid three-legged stool. I didn't whistle and sing anymore.

My only recourse was to join the navy as soon as I was of age. Nevertheless, when I returned from the great wars that same old stupid cow, her milk, the milk bucket and stool were waiting for me just as I left it. I prayed fervently, "O Lord, I'm really a good boy—lift this horrible burden from me and give it back to my sister, and I will be eternally thankful." Like my Dad, the Lord said, "No."

Most significantly, though, the one bit of discernment I gained from my cow milking experience was the poignant meaning of the 10th Commandment. "Thou shalt not covet." In time I discovered that it's okay to pursue success and things that make for happiness and fulfillment. But when the want becomes so excessive that it evolves into lust, sits on our front burner all the time, and drives us to do the wrong, then it is covetousness, and that is sin, and we need to be cognizant of that quite early.

So, take an old sage's advice, practice unselfishness and kindness—otherwise, you might find yourself milking a cow twice a day, every day, or joining the navy.

LIGHTS AND PIGS

I love lights—I switch them on in every room. What's more, I don't turn them off. Because of that my wife calls me names like compulsive, disorderly and psychoparanoia. Unremittingly, she stays on my case regarding my peculiar conduct. But I simply must have lights—all about me, and I'll tell you why.

The most ego boosting distinction in my high school days was to have a girlfriend in another town not your own. Next, was to have transportation. Luckily, I had both.

In my case, it was Dad's combination feed and chicken truck to make social calls on. Because of my good fortune in these area's my male peers—seemingly—looked upon me as someone of maturity and experiencing a little more of life than they.

Consequently, I transmuted comfortably into that mold. I, indeed, walked with aloofness among my fellas—saying little of my esoterical romance in that distant community. And its value multiplied exceedingly.

But two major problems plagued Dad's pickup. The left rear fender was split in half leaving the divided portions hanging loosely—thus creating a loud clanging noise when the vehicle was in motion.

Next was the unpleasant odors from live poultry and animal feeds that emanated from the auto like a wet stock pen. Needless to say, my motored conveyance constituted a significant embarrassment to me when visiting my girl.

It was a lovely summer evening that I was to take my date out on an extra special occasion.

I felt my attire exceptionally appropriate. I wore overly starched, white trousers that made slicing sounds when walking, and a long-sleeved, cotton shirt turned up neatly at the cuffs. As was the custom, my hair was watered down with four ounces of scented Brilliantine—parted in the middle, and combed back smooth as a shoe shine. In the mirror I was simply too wonderful to behold.

By no means, though, would I drive Dad's noisy—smelly rig to my girlfriend's home. So I parked it in front of the post office and started walking the three blocks on the sidewalk to her house. There were no street lights and the night was dark.

Unfortunately, no one told me the sidewalk went just so far. And how was I to know that where it ended, a muddy, hog wallow began?

Perky, and in high spirits—and whistling a sprightly tune I stepped off the pavement onto the back of a reposing sow and her nursing piglets. Immediately, a cacophony of squeals, grunts and snorts erupted into unleashed pandemonium, and I felt myself catapulted upward and suspended momentarily between heaven and quagmire.

Then down I came—tumbling topsy-turvy—all of me—slicing trousers and sleeves turned up neatly at the cuff. SPLAT! Indeed, what was anticipated to be a delightful outing ended unexpectedly simply because of lack of light.

Against this backdrop, I respond to my mate's scolding when I'm caught in my turn-them-all-on mania. "Dear, you are just flat out wrong," I argue. "I certainly have no mental disorders—it's just … well, ah, well … I just don't want to step on another hog. Can't you understand that?"

More seriously, even a little light at times can be priceless. But people should also value moral and spiritual light as well as natural illumination. God is light and without His enlightenment to humankind, evil leads at will.

The Creator has given the world, His Holy Spirit, the Bible and the church to give energy and comprehension of His luminosity. If this is not true, how else would persons know where the good walkways of this life end and the swine mires begin? So let His radiant mind guide you daily.

SHELLBACKS AND POLLIWOGS

A large decorative document from World War II hangs on my bedroom wall. Within its frame, beautiful mermaids ride great fish side saddle beneath the boisterous swells ... cavorting with myriad creatures of the deep.

In its backdrop—crowned King Neptune and his four white stallions rise out of the tumultuous sea. On this treasured certificate of mine is written these privileged words:

"To all sailors where ever ye may be: Be it remembered that Joseph E. Fulford (me) having been found worthy to be numbered as one of our trusty Shellbacks has been duly initiated into the solemn mysteries of the Ancient Order of the Deep." Signed, Neptunus Rex, Ruler of the Raging Main.

More than likely, under U.S. Navy tradition a sailor becomes a Shellback while crossing the equator and undergoing the prescribed initiation. Before that transpires, however, the seaman is simply a lower than low polliwog, and will thus remain until crossing the earth's midriff and duly admitted into the Shellback order.

On my ship two thirds of the crew, including me, had never been near the equator, and, therefore, held the ignoble distinction of being despicable polliwogs. That status was soon to change, though. Our ship, at that moment, was plying due South—enroute to a remote pacific island lying below the equator which we were soon to cross.

We nothings, admittedly—approached the world's middle with little or no apprehension of the so called Passover rites ... just more Navy Scuttlebut. What's more, we didn't know or care that the crossing ceremonies would last two days beginning the day before we actually traversed the earth's middle—so what.

But on the first day a major metamorphosis set in among some of the, otherwise, good ole boys. It became quite obvious that an adversarial change was rapidly occurring on the ship. Our Shellback mates quickly discarded their shirts revealing pirate's scull and crossbones glaring menacingly from their chests. With bandannas tied around their foreheads they began sorely harassing the polliwog populace.

The Shellbacks heckled us at every turn. Mates on their hit list woke up with the dreaded scull and crossbones stenciled on their brows, indicating severe retribution awaited them. Even tough old polliwog salts turned jittery and glazy.

Extreme anxiety, needless to say, quickly spilled into the ship's polliwog company, and we of the crew's unregenerate subculture could not peep out a hatchway without having our heads slammed by a jet of water from full throttle fire hoses.

The Shellbacks, in addition, made stocks to fasten worthless one's heads and hands in—welded them to the deck and filled them with captives and stuffed ice into the hapless victim's pockets.

Little imagination was needed to fathom what naked ice, against the skin, feels like when unremoved. So like field rabbits, we polliwogs sought hiding places and were real quiet and still, hoping to escape the marauding Shellbacks, but they, like hunting hounds, sniffed us out.

Then unexpectedly, in the midst of the melee, an illuminated polliwog shrieked, "Hey! There's a lot more of us than them." The revelation caught hold and quickly traveled the length and breadth of the ship.

A mob like frenzy seized us as we easily captured some fire hoses and turned them on our oppressors and sent squealing Shellbacks skidding, helter-skelter, down the deck in delightful blasts of sweet, vengeful water spurts.

Snorting victory, we ripped up the stocks—freed the subjugated, and tossed the mess into the sea. We took some prisoners ourselves and cuffed them around a bit. They pleaded for mercy, but good fellow feeling was not on our agenda that day.

Doubtless, the honey sweetness of punishing had arrested our souls, and we were giddy with power and success, and demonstrated it to the utmost on the outnumbered Shellbacks.

Oddly enough, though, I don't think any polliwog ascertained, at the moment, that the next day our ship would pass over the equator, and, then, it would become mandatory we submit to the traditional initiation rites at the hands of these same Shellbacks we were so happily punishing.

The attack came at dawn. With fiery vengeance fixed in their eyes and belching smoke and flame the Shellbacks took absolute control. By command, the polliwog dress on that fateful day was trousers only ... nothing else.

Barefoot, and lined up like columns of POW's on the steel deck, rubber shoed Shellbacks splashed us with water from fire hoses. Sharp discharges of electricity on the metal flooring kept us squirming and dancing. As expected, each polliwog must stand alone before his majesty, King Neptune, to face charges—be judged, sentenced—punished.

But prior to courtly proceedings the polliwog must first partake of the royal fruit (onions soaked in castor oil) and kiss the belly of the king's baby (a five foot six, 250 pound sweaty Shellback with black motor grease and dirt rubbed on his stomach).

The Monarch's dreaded belt line followed next, without delay. The walloping pieces weren't your average waist line belts, but cut sections of fire hoses soaked in sea water—flattened and dried. Twenty "eye for eye, tooth for tooth" freebooters faced each other with salt hardened straps ready.

By the time I tasted Neptune's oily delicacy I had had enough, I lost it—that is, I mutated rapidly into one hundred twenty-seven pounds of spindly rage. I snarled and spit the greasy onion into the face of the royal baby. But before I could voice my pent-up indignation, I was swatted down on my hands and knees between those primed straps.

Two solid whacks sent my skinny body skiing across the deck amidst strident laughter along with more swats. Two chortling pirates snatched me up like three pounds of chicken and I stood face-to-face before the ruler of the raging main, perched on his throne.

His highness charged me with lubricating the ship's rigging with ten cent jars of Vaseline, and through it all I was hopping and skipping from burst's of electric current in the deck while constantly ordered to stand still or face contempt of court.

The verdict was guilty. My penalty: undergo royal surgery and receive a stately haircut to bring me in line and enhance self esteem. Kingly physicians were at the ready with saw, hammers, and screwdrivers. I felt my thin body pitched onto a table where a sudden jolt of current lit up my hip bones and toes.

Then, without warning, I was haphazardly tossed up onto a high platform, with chair, to sustain the Ocean Potentate's ordered head crop. Twenty feet below me sat one of our landing boats filled to the brim with water. Inside it stood three scruffy, Shellback buccaneers.

"Just a trim," I said, as the clippers cut a three inch swath across the top of my head from ear to ear. Then, from the forehead to the nape of the neck—leaving four little islet's of hair on my mutilated pate.

"Tonic?" the king's barber asked, as he lathered my noggin with "can't wash out" black tar liquid using a paint brush. Before I could do serious damage to this hair butcher the chair tipped over and I plummeted into the water below.

Just as quickly the Shellbacks swept me up and howled in my face, "What are you?"

"Polliwog," I sputtered. Back under the water I went. Then up again. "What are you?" they shouted again. A light came on, "Shellback!" I yelled, "Shellback!" then they smiled, laughed, shook my hand—bear hugged me and set me on a dry, tranquil foundation and made me a bonafide member of the Shellback brotherhood.

Let me say that since that long ago Navy experience I have passed through another indoctrination rite vastly different and more consequential than my introduction into the Royal Order of Shellbacks.

It was, of course, my inception into the kingdom of God whose citizens enjoy far better rewards than an ancient document hanging on the bedroom wall.

The Prince of the bounteous life is clear about first steps into his province. He would say, if you want a better—more peaceful, productive life. If you desire an existence where forgiveness is a must … a comfort zone where a body can relax, sleep contentedly, function properly and digest food appropriately. If you covet an assurance of the forever presence of you maker, less anxiety and his unseen angels to watch over you; then you must take the initial step. You must "first seek the kingdom of God and his righteousness and all things needful (and much more) shall be added unto you" (Matt. 6:33).

In the process of the induction into God's realm you must believe with all your mind that God is a can-do power and loves you with all his heart, with a love bond that cannot be broken.

So begin working to clear your conscience of guilt and bad habits by conferring your weakness and wrong ways to God. Let repentance take your life in another direction. And by all means get a new attitude—mirror God's love in you to others, even your enemies. And when you complete the master's acceptance contract—Baptism, let it be with joy and excitement.

Walk in faith as a subject of God's country on earth and you will have entered that province of a chosen generation and you shall learn the secret of full measure living now and a forever life to come. Hang it in your heart and not on the wall.

DUMB YANKEE

In a glass case in the living room my wife displays memorabilia from the two World Wars. There is a 1917 picture of her uncle and some of his postcards from Paris. Beside that are pictures of her brother and me in our navy blues. I remember those days well. At the time I was a seventeen-year old—five foot eleven—a one hundred thirty-five pound, bonafide son of the South eager to enlist and wrap up World War II in short order.

My friend, Bob, and I, along with a gaggle of other recruits, boarded the train for Jacksonville to be duly sworn into the U.S. Navy. We both had fifteen dollars each to last until payday. Now, freed from the inhibiting shackles of home rules we openly smoked cigarettes—blew smoke rings—used some profanity—talked and giggled, and looked out the train window with the joyful abandonment of the newly liberated ... how wonderful it was.

As the train rocked and rumbled, squeaked and squilled us to our great destiny a service man, with an up-north accent and lots of colored medals on his khaki shirt, paused at our seats to chat awhile. I listened to his nasal "cheeze" and "for Christ sakes" a few moments and thought to myself—"dumb Yankee."

But the soldier was warm and friendly and said he saw us get on the train at Marianna and presumed we were navy recruits on our way to Jacksonville. He thought it really great, young boys like us joining up to fight for our great country and even give our lives if necessary. I began to soften. Then he said, "Cheeze, you good looking guys want to play some cards—kill a little time?"

Five minutes later he left us with a sagging, hangdog countenance and thirty dollars poorer. Paralyzed and dumbfounded, I heard the dumb Yankee's obliging intonation further down the aisle to some up-town fella's like Bob and me, "Cheeze, you good looking guys want to play some cards—kill a little time?

Boot camp was laden with unpleasant surprises. One especially was the humongous drillfield and some hard lessons on how to march on it while staying in lock step with multitudes all around you. Morning—afternoon—and many times at night we tramped to the cadence call of our company officer (CO) "yer lep—yer lep—yer lep right lep—follow you lep—hup, hup, hup, ri ... hup ..."

Relentlessly, our CO strove to mold us on that field, and within a few weeks we had actually graduated to marching with a mock rifle on our shoulders correctly. But shoot, I already knew how to walk with a gun. I'd hunted squirrels enough to know that. Fact is, to carry a gun properly just rest it sideways on the shoulder muscle with the barrel leaning against the back of the neck. It's the way Dad did it.

Even so, I at once heard this agitated bellow as we marched, "Straighten that rifle you nitwit!" Then the same urgent request came again accompanied with some unprintable words, and I thought to myself, "some dumb Yankee kid don't know how to carry a rifle."

But seconds later the CO raced down those moving ranks to where I was and came near breaking my neck as he adjusted my rifle for me. From that day forth I, indeed, bore my rifle in a military fashion, so called—not like my Dad did.

On top of that, I didn't realize I wasn't staying in step with my mates on the drill field either. When the CO said "Lep" my left foot wasn't altogether on the ground—but close enough not to make any difference. And besides, who would ever notice a thing like that with all those moving feet and legs around me? So I let it go at that—who cared?

But then I heard that ungentle shout again, "get in step you ...!" Don't make me come in there ...!" Again I thought, "this time for sure, it's some dumb Yankee kid out of step—boy, will he ever get it. I'd hate to be in his shoes."

I had not quite absorbed my innocent cognition when the CO pounced on me and had me bouncing off the pavement while leading me through the skipping procedure to get my "lep" down on lep time.

So even today when my wife and I take our walks I try to stay in step with her while calling cadence, "you lep—you lep—ri, lep!" No, I'm not crazy I tell her, I just don't want to be yanked around any more.

The wonder of it all, though, was that by the end of boot camp the dumb Yankees and the sons of the South were marching together as one—every rifle straight—every foot in step—even mine. It was gratifying to be a part of it and feel good about my Yankee brothers. They weren't so dumb after all.

But today throngs, indeed, are out of step with God. Like the cadence call of my ancient CO, our maker is calling us to align ourselves with Him and get in step with His ways. To walk to the beat of our Creator brings peace and harmony to the soul and one another and makes every day brighter.

So, my sisters and brothers, get in step with the Lord of heaven and earth, or like my long ago CO, He might go in there where you are and make the necessary adjustments and that would be grievous.

GOD, SOAP POWDER AND CHINCH BUGS

Back when an economy size box of Tide washing powder was thirty nine cents and the price of an annual lawn spraying was $14.00, my wife and I struggled to keep up with the Jones' in yard care. Healthy grasses and shrubbery were status symbols in our neighborhood and we simply wanted to stay on par with our friends.

But $14.00 was a lot of money in those lean times. What's more, there was the watering—fertilizing—cutting, adinfinitum. Our yard upkeep, simply put, had a prodigious impact on our meager budget.

To hold down cost, though, I persisted aggressively with our grassy plot. I cut—trimmed—watered—created a compost pile, and clubbed giant grasshoppers with my hoe handle; and unknown to my wife, I made two pieces of lengthy caterpillars with her sewing scissors. In short, I labored with vigor and inventiveness to make our domicile as attractive as our neighbor's.

But all that work had no effect on those grass killing chinch bugs. Every year, with voracious appetites they attacked our precious herbage. Come spring, I would notice a section of our lawn turning pale—then widen into a drab brown and I knew I had to scrape up $14.00 to pay the spray man. At the time $14.00 bought a week's supply of groceries and even gas for the car.

Serendipities, however, will often come to those with sharp ears and keen minds, so I listened judiciously to a sagacious voice proffering sage like tidings on how to eradicate chinch bugs without dishing out all that money.

"You can rid yourself of those bugs for less than two bucks," the voice intoned.

Immediately, my interest leaped from the back to the front burner. "How?"

"A piece of cake," the voice continued. "Get three thirty-nine cent economy size boxes of Tide—sprinkle the contents evenly over the lawn—water down with hose until your yard is covered with white suds—let it soak in overnight—results—dead and dying chinch bugs. Cost—zilch." Glory!

It was with exuberant eagerness, indeed, that my wife and I followed the Tide formula to the letter. Before dusk our yard appeared as if a foot of summer snow had fallen. The frothy foam popped, bubbled and fizzed over our entire tract. And from that burbling effervescence I could hear those dirty little critters—pleading for their lives ... gasping for breath. Fittingly a sinister chuckle issued from my lips as I quietly mused, "die—die—you filthy Blisses Leucopterus ... Receive your just deserts." Chuckle, chuckle.

Actually, I'd just as soon cut this off right here, but my cognitation tells me this whole episode howls for an answer to the burning question ... did it work? NO, NO, NO, it didn't work. In fact, the brown places grew larger by the day until I finally called the exterminator.

Right away he wanted to know why I hadn't called earlier. So, with a shrug of the shoulders and abashed countenance I hemmed and hawed striving desperately to banish the spreading pink on my cheeks. Finally, I timorously confessed the soap powder treatment.

My pest control man gave me a long dead-pan look. Then he smiled—and laughed ... he laughed some more—and in the process he became hysterical. At last, between spasms, he managed to say, "you folks may not have dead chinch bugs, but I'm willing to bet you've got the most sanitized ones in town." More laughter. I paid him $14.00.

Similarly, the religious life, like my chinch bug experience, can come up peculiarly lacking at times. Far too often even the faithful endeavor to seek other ways rather than the tried and true—and what a messy mess falls into their laps.

Many, like myself, get snared in various winds of wrong approaches. We covet social status—prestige and prominence, not to mention an inordinate passion for beautiful homes and cars—correct friends and lots of money. To have these things are not sins. Our enigma, however, is that all too frequently our Creator is bypassed in the fervent press for the good life.

The soap powder and chinch bugs mentality simply doesn't lessen the myriad pesty beasts in human behavior. But God can. He can remove logs from eyes and cobwebs from brains and set aright. He will give the Spirit of discernment to those who ask. Why not read His book and learn of Him and give His way a try. It's free.

I'M NO FOOT WASHER

There are encounters in life—both physical and emotional—that are so poignant and often dissimilar, but, yet, are forever etched in the mind's memory bank. Let me tell you of two of mine. I begin first—with nature's human extremities.

My wife—without question, was a passionate foot washer. So was my mother. Both, apparently, were hopelessly obsessed with dirty foot phobia and had rather endure horrible misfortune than be caught themselves, or their household, with the slightest tint of grime on either foot ... especially at bedtime.

Moreover, their cogent tidings to humanity was ... if you want a better world, then begin by scrubbing spotless your toes, ankles and all in between.

I've always had a sneaking suspicion, too, that these two fixated ladies quietly tiptoed throughout the house at night with flashlights checking their offspring's feet. Fact is, even my dad—regal head of the domicile, wasn't excluded from this intrusion.

They, indeed, stood by the sage pronouncement: if feet were washed until the skin flashed, then the soul took note and was quieted and comforted and gave the whole body a night of guilt-free slumber. Thus, according to this doctrine, man had been well served and God was pleased and smiling.

As for me, though, I harbor no sentiments concerning clean or unclean feet. Wash or don't is okay by me. Unlike my helpmeet and my mom, I don't think God does either.

So I turned the corner long ago and happily told the world that I'm no foot washer and I lay bare why I made the decision and why my recall is so striking. So you be the judge of my resolve.

If you've ever, per chance, been forced out of a warm bed on a polar, cold night—driven to the back porch bare foot under extreme coercion, drawn a bucket of ice water from a deep well ... poured it into a frozen, galvanized tin tub and plunged your feet in just to make them unsullied again, then you can understand my acute, adverse feelings toward foot washing and why its frigid memory scatters chill bumps liberally over my skin.

Similarly graphic but tender is the emotional experience.

There was, in one of my parishes an elderly couple. Both are in heaven now, but I will remember them as long as I live because they opened to view deep feelings of compassion in their hearts at its loveliest.

They drove an ancient Hudson—lived off a small, monthly, social security check—paid their tithes and never missed a church service or prayer meeting.

I can still see them at the Bible study—him wearing little bird-egg glasses on the end of his nose sitting next to his wife with her great shock of white hair—sharing with him the Bible in her lap. There was, tellingly, a pronounced enthrallment on their faces when the scriptures were read and discussed.

Then the Church had an urgent four week's drive to raise money for our World Service and Conference Benevolence to feed the hungry. At the end of the month this dear lady gave me seven dollars in quarters tied up in a wrinkled handkerchief to send to our mission project. She said she and her husband had decided to do without some food and give the money to those hungry people.

I simply could not speak. These two old saints, barely existing on their meager livelihood—paying their bills and tithes out of that, and now, taking more from it to help others. I found a private place and wept.

These two angels are forever engrafted in my conscious, and I humbly bow my head and say with Peter, "Lord wash not my feet only, but also my hands and my head" (John 13:9). Even with ice cold well water if it will give me a heart like theirs.

NIGHT OF THE SNAKE

I once possessed a full measure of Sigmund Freud's ID, Ego and Super Ego—but it wasn't all my fault—my wife and kids were much to blame. Had I not heard my spouse, many times, describe me as the bravest person she had ever known?

And didn't she tell our friends how safe and secure she felt with me? And our two little girls have said in my hearing that even Gunsmoke's great Matt Dillon was no match for their dad.

Needless to say, I reveled in their plaudits, and right early began walking with an air of intrepidness and speaking with firm demeanor. My only problem, however, was that my fortitude was untested. But that was soon to come.

Our abode was a little white cottage with a front porch in a wooded area that could only be approached over a two-rutted dirt road. An ancient water oak sheltered the verandah. As it was, we had spent the weekend with my parents and returned late Sunday evening in a deluge of wind and rain.

Fortunately, the inclement weather had subsided some on our arrival. The headlights clearly lit up the portico, but the windgusts had caused a branch from the oak to break and fall on the porch roof. It was a twisted bough with the greater part curving under the overhang—almost reaching the door.

Nothing exciting about that except the oversized black snake coiled around the detached limb flicking his tongue grotesquely in the car lights. Obviously, an instinctive foreboding seized my family. In short, they weren't about to get out of the car with that dragon at the door.

But I knew the serpent was harmless and began to perceive this as my moment—a serendipity to play out for all its worth. Now was the time for my family to observe—first hand—the fearless head-of-the-house in action.

"Don't be frightened," I assured them in take-charge tone. "Ole daddy-o will handle this."

Cavalierly, I got out of the car and found a good solid stick. Planning ahead I hypothesized how best to dislodge the snake and further embellish my lion-hearted image.

First, I would give the reptile a firm whack, knocking him to the floor. Then I would crouch and pounce on the beast—grab him behind his head—briefly struggle with his writhing body—pretend the thing was dead, then toss him into the bushes where he would crawl for his life.

Afterward, I assumed, my wife and children would fall at my feet and do homage. Glory! My id-Ego and super Ego were feasting sumptuously at this resplendent banquet. O, what joy comes to those who work at it.

Undaunted, I swung my weapon with all my might, but I missed the animal and impacted the branch with such force that it unhinged and shoved itself and the lapping tongue within inches of my face.

An uncontrollable, squealy sound issued from my throat as I tumbled backward over two rocking chairs onto the ground. But the snake kept a coming. I howled and thrashed around in the dirt and wet leaves like someone on fire.

Albeit, my wife—manifesting awesome courage—ran over with the umbrella and chased the creature away. Later, in quieted shame and down-cast countenance I made a pact with my spouse and girls to never, no, never, say nothing to nobody about Daddy-o's night with the snake.

"We live in dangerous times," is a much used cliché. And, indeed, we do. Undeniably, there is a universal breakdown in the perception of right and wrong. But have you ever wondered why?

Here is something to consider. An ancient apostle declares the basic reason for immorality and violence is that persons are inordinate "lovers of themselves" (2 Tim. 3:2 ff.).

By any measure, excessive self-admiration evolves into a variety of spiritual and moral maladies that eventually culminate in insatiable lust and savagery.

Such is humanity's daily meat. Indeed, before one horror passes another overlaps and takes its place. And because of the constant overfamiliarity with these things it has become even more tolerable with today's citizenry. But to God it's all destructive sin—delivering nothing but heartbreak and disappointment.

False pride does not come from heaven, but humility does. Doubtless, hazardous years lie ahead for humankind. But let us proceed with all of God's requisites stored in our hearts.

And what are His family rules? "He hath shown thee, o man, what is good ... to do justly, and to love mercy, and to walk humbly with thy God" (Micha 6:8).

So let God see your humility everyday, or you, too, might find a snake on the porch some stormy night, or worse.

CAST NETS AND ANGELS

A cast net is used to catch more than one fish at a time, and can be managed by a single person. They come in various sizes—say—from six to twelve feet in diameter when spread out. In particular, if thrown properly the larger one will cover an area of water the size of a large room.

Indisputably, though, beginning netters with no basic skills should begin with a junior net until some throwing experience is acquired. Unfortunately, the only net I could borrow to learn the art was of the mega strain—preferred by professionals.

"Big fish rig like that—no problem for you," a netter friend assured me. "You're tall. Here, let me show you how easy it is."

Proficiently, my tutor demonstrated how to first fold the meshes over the right arm in layers leaving just enough in the left hand to heave, and how to loop the tether around the wrist. Then he put one of the lead weights skirting the meshwork edges between his teeth.

"Holding a lead sinker in the mouth," he pointed out, "keeps the webbing from bunching when thrown ... Now—watch me."

He stood firmly—legs apart—and turned his body slightly to the right. Then with pronounced force he swung back—masterly launching the twelve footer with impressive might and artistry.

The net whirled out before him—rapidly playing off his arm and dropped a perfect circle into the water. That done my teacher explained how the leads sank first and fast—pulling the net down and together, entrapping the unwary fish.

Golly, gee, I must learn to do that. So jumping right in I eagerly began my modus operandi, but promptly met a complication. For the life of me I couldn't remember to let the sinker between my teeth go at the right time, and I had no teeth to spare.

"No big deal," my instructor promised. "Just get yourself a clothes pin—tie it around your neck with a stout cord and fasten one of the leads in it. When you throw, the jerk of the net will pop it right out."

My wife and I had two little girls—two and six. Since we lived near the Gulf of Mexico we took them to the beach most every summer afternoon after work. These outings turned out to be an opportune time to practice my new hobby off the pier while my spouse watched the children on the shore.

But my six year old sensed my excitement and insisted on accompanying me on the dock. So with clothespin tied firmly around my neck I clamped the meshwork over my right arm as instructed. At the time, I didn't know a brand new clothespin with a metal spring clipped just right could potentially lift a large man off the floor.

I told my daughter to stand back while I made the cast. Wow! Like magic the net twirled out a flawless disc before me.

Unblemished it was—that is—until it met the lead weight in the clothespin, and there it abruptly stopped.

As the sheer heaviness of the contraption whisked my body over the safety rail I clasped the top bar with both hands and held on with all my strength.

In short, there I was—legs up—head down—faintly calling out in frantic desperation—help, help. The fish netting still held intact by the clothespin appeared to pour out of my mouth for twelve feet down. My little girl, peering at my face through the guard slats asked excitedly, "Daddy, did you catch a big one?"

As I looked down at the undulating, blue-green sea I could hear running feet and frenzied voices, "hurry, grab him, quick … he's going over." Many hands clutched my legs and arms and pulled me back to safety.

Stunned and discountenanced I watched my rescuers haul in my borrowed net—disconnect it from the clothespin and set me free. Well, was I lucky that day or was it something more?

Indeed, I believe God has appointed a guardian angel to each person to provide providential care, or else there would be few, if any overcomers—especially me. Does not the Holy writ expressly describe angels as,

"Are they not all ministering spirits, sent forth to minister for them who shall be heirs of salvation?" (Hebrews 1:14). By all means, every human should tap into that.

Later, my call was to be a minister. But I feel certain my angel—while protecting me from fishing mishaps and other things—must have inquired of the Father time and time again if He was quite certain I was the right one to be a fisher of men.

Fortunately for persons, the captain of souls gives up on no one. "Lo, I am with you always, even unto the end of the age" (Matt. 28:20). He promises.

So get in touch with heaven and claim your angel. They are more real than you think. By the way, stay away from big cast nets.

THE SAFETY VALVE

In those good old days my weekly salary was a whopping forty-eight dollars before taxes—straight pay—long hours. Even with some belt tightening, my wife and two little girls—six and two, barely made do until payday next. Needless to say, our meager cash flow patently confined our range of recreation to the radio, a now-and-then movie at the drive-in and rocking on the front porch.

I also drove an ailing forty-six Ford with a slow leak in the left rear tire. No big deal, though, after all, I had a tire pump in the trunk. But the battery was another angst altogether. The poor thing was old and feeble and suffered terribly from congestive cell failure. Doubtless, its terminal affliction was becoming more apparent each day.

But to keep our budget balanced I had to squeeze as much life out of it as possible. My redress, however, to its malady was to hang my yard sale, battery booster on a tree next to the car—raise the hood—clip on the IV's and switch on the current. Those precious life lines kept the battery alive overnight and provided the energy to crank and run the auto the next day.

Fortunately, my charger was portable, so it, too, rode in the rear beside the air pump when not in use.

But to leave the house on any given night was, indeed, a total disregard to all prudence. Of course, that's precisely what we did when we piled our two kids into our impaired heap along with a coke bottle of kerosene for mosquito repellent—a jug of ice tea, some cheese and saltine crackers and headed for the open air movies.

After parking and placing the speaker on the door I threaded the air hose onto the valve stem of the slow leaker, and connected the charger to the battery. After the show I'd hop out—quickly pump up the tire—detach from the valve stem—crank up—disconnect the booster and be off as smooth as a table top.

Now, against this backdrop, my wife and I were invited, one evening, to a cookware party at a neighbor's home. We were among a selected few, so our host said, to observe, first hand, a complementary meal prepared for us in the most current state-of-the-art pressure cooker. Free supper? Yes! We went.

After dinner, the introduction, predictably, was a sales pitch to sell the amazing utensil—and there it sat proudly on the stove, having done its job superbly. It was a gorgeous thing and shiny as a brand new truck.

Impressive, high tech accessories adorned its cover ... a turn knob to tighten it onto the main pot—a chimney like steam whistle to release pressure and a glass tube marked with scaled numbers with a bubble inside to gauge compaction.

Then there was the safety valve. "But," assured the salesman, "for precautionary purposes only. In fact, no attachments to provide safeguards on any of our products have ever been known to blow—ever."

Moreover, he continued. One of the most valued benefits in owning one of these machines was social. It was no secret. Your status in the neighborhood will soar—folks will simply envy you—you will be somebody, and your self-esteem will go through the roof. And if there are lingering doubts among you our company will supply you with dozens of testimonies from happy satisfied customers.

Just think, this magnificent mechanism takes less cooking time than ordinary stoveware, and holds the unrivaled reputation of allowing no vitamins or nutrients to escape the food.

"Dear friends," he opined. "After feasting from this mechanical breakthrough a few weeks you will feel better—sleep sounder—have a sweeter disposition and unlimited vitality. What's more, you can have this fabulous appliance for a limited time only—for the incredible give-away price of sixty dollars—payable with only two dollars down and one dollar a week."

Wow! My wife nodded her approval and I plopped down two bucks while the man wrote the order. Three days later we happily put our regal implement on the stove. Truly it was a prestige piece and maybe someday a collector's item. We breathed proud, my wife and I.

When not in use, we kept the precious thing polished and in sight for friends and neighbors to see. Indeed, our most gratifying delight was for someone to say to us, "you folks must be filthy rich to own a kettle like that." Ah, it was so pleasant to be somebody.

At the time there was playing at the drive in a must-see film about armies of rampaging, killer ants in South America. We just simply could not miss that thriller.

Our agenda, as usual, was for my family to eat early. I, in turn, would rush home from work, grab a bite, load us up and beeline it to the picture show.

But that afternoon my wife decided to try her hand at cooking some dried, Great Northern beans in our brand new, time saver appliance. A big mistake, because when I arrived home I quickly discovered that the Titanic had sunk, meaning, the safety valve on our invincible utensil had exploded.

From any strategic point of view Yankee legumes had blasted the south. They were everywhere—on the ceiling, stove, walls, floor, curtains. Correctly, my wife characterized our infallible cooker as abruptly metamorphosing into a loose machine gun with a stuck trigger that wouldn't stop until every bean-bullet was fired.

Furthermore, our six year old, in her effort to help mom clean up, had blistered her hand good on hot beans. She was soaking it in a pan of cold water. Boy-o-boy, was my wife ever piqued.

Under the circumstance we backed off and decided to forego the ants that evening. But our scorched daughter would have none of that. She wept and whaled and had an answer for every alibi we could think of.

She would help clean the kitchen … Her hand didn't hurt that bad anymore—and besides, she could take along the pan of water, just in case, and we wouldn't have to bother with cheese and crackers and ice tea.

We weakened under her persuasive lamentation and determined to try it one more time. The kids went to the living room while their mother and I cleaned up the beans. It was a summer and the floor fan was on. Suddenly, we heard a dull flutter from the fan and a high pitched bawl from our oldest.

Rushing to the scene we discovered our daughter had playfully squeezed her cute little toes through the fan guard and into the whirling blades. Thankfully, no toes were missing or skin broken. And we concluded that after all we'd been through the killer ants would afford us a relaxing diversion. So we made ready—kerosene, ice tea, cheese, crackers and a pan of cold water just in case.

Out the door we went toward our reposing jalopy. There it sat—hood up, with two cables dropping under it from the charger fastened to the trees. Something wasn't quite right, though, and a sinking feeling washed over my liver. One of the lines had come loose from the battery.

Anxiously, I jumped into the car and turned the starter ... row,row,row. Again, row, row. Again—click. Dead. That did it. No ants for us that night and I wanted to scream my rage at the high heavens. Fact is, I nearly lost my sense of humor. Truly, I thought, all things work together for the bad ...

But later in life, in my struggle to discern why the wrong, all too often, prevails over the right and good, I reread the Bible verse, "man that is born of woman is of few days, and full of trouble" (Job 14:1). Frankly, I had been quite skeptical of that statement. But after the pressure cooker and car experience I was out-and-out convinced of its reality.

Furthermore, I simply assumed providence had singled me out for amusement purposes. On the contrary, however, I discovered personal travails are universal. They are the property of everyone. Daily tensions and pressures are there—they are real and must be mollified lest the sparks of misery get locked in.

These distresses, fortunately, can be lessened because the human is equipped to overcome or modify the adverse.

Some therapists suggest taking time periodically, to do good deeds for the less fortunate. And that is excellent therapy.

Others advise responding to the invitation of the Great Physician to come to Him and talk it over in the privacy of His unseen office, "And find rest unto your souls" (Matt. 11:29B). Great anxiety reducing benefits here.

Another method is what Holy writ defines as "edifying one another" (1 Thess. 5:11). This approach calls for a particular kind of encouraging dialogue interchanged with fellow women and men. The sweet relief comes when burdens are shared, when prayers are given and a hand or shoulder is touched in friendship. There is, indeed, healing elements in such fellowship.

In such a gathering the spirit of Love courses through each one giving strength and motivation to stay in the game of life. Consequently, existence, with all its perplexities becomes much less threatening.

I recall a little girl, some years back, during my children's sermon on the importance of "Quietness." "But Pastor," she said, "I can't be quiet all the time, cause things just build up inside so bad I just gotta get them out—then they're not so bad anymore."

How profound, get it out, talk to someone about it, don't hold it in until it explodes like our pressure cooker filled with Great Northern beans. You'll be glad you did.

MY VERY OWN WORD

Some time ago I read, or heard, a rather unconventional technique on how to become a masterful, sought after conversationalist. The way to improve your dialogue—so the concept goes—is to first pay close attention to unfamiliar words in your reading that are usually passed over. Sooner or later you will discover an unknown word that you like.

To me, the interpretation of that idea, was to make that singular word your very own; fall in love with it. In other words, let yourself and the word become one. Repeat it over and over until it becomes a melody in your heart. But never, no, never, look up or ask for the meaning of the word. Such knowledge would surely diminish the joy of its usage. And then, when you become familiar enough with your word, begin sprinkling it into your conversation. Chances are your hearers won't know the meaning either. But they will certainly think your gentile qualities exceptionally polished.

Indeed, I thought this a fantastic insight—it was definitely worth a try. So I began keeping a watchful eye for that special word I could claim. Then one day I chanced upon the word "redundant." Instantly I knew that was it. The word just reached out and embraced me. Indeed, it held a sweet savory sound of refinement and sparkle as we bonded. There it lay, a symbol of beauty in a string of plain common words. It, of course, was love at first sight and I wondered why such a nice word like "redundant" was nixed in with old every day, ordinary words. I would rescue this eloquent locution and make it mine.

From that moment on I spent time repeating the word over and over. I would even sing it to myself—re-dun-dant, re-dun-dant; re-dun-re-dun-reda-da-dant, fitting it into most any tune. It was a love affair with us two—the word and I.

And very soon I began indulging it in my dialogue with others. I inserted it extravagantly by voice on every occasion for descriptive phrases and explanations on any subject. Delicious food tasted redundant—facial expressions were redundant. How do you feel? Well, I feel a little redundant this morning. Occasionally, I detected a lifted eyebrow and puzzled looks on my listeners, quick-glancing one another. But, shoot—it's my word and they were jealous because they couldn't use such a beautiful word like I could.

Furthermore, the word was serving me well and I used it lavishly … that is, until I went to college at a late age. O Mercy me, it simply had to happen. I had written a four-page essay for a class project and got my daughter, also a college student, to type it for me. A few days later my graded paper was returned and I eagerly opened it to see my grade and the professor's comments. Would you believe it? There was my very own word "redundant" written to the side of each paragraph on all four pages. Wow! A feeling of exhilaration surged through my bones. My instructor was surely a friend of my word. I liked that.

Later I saw my daughter and she was eager to know what grade I received on my essay. As proud as I could be, I handed her the paper—lifting my chest in glory and victoriously voiced, "I made a 'redundant' grade." She looked at the paper and squealed with laughter and asked, "Dad, do you know what redundant means?" Silly question. "Sure, I know what redundant means—it means something so incomparable that no other word could match it—not in a million years."

"Wrong, Dad. Redundant means too many words. Your paper is too wordy, wordy. Dad, you ought to look these words up in the dictionary." Well, I was jolted, to say the least, but I did look up the word, reluctantly, and my heart sank as the mask was peeled from my sweet word exposing it for what it really was—too many words, in my case, and not much else.

Well, I must confess I used a lot of hyperbole in regards to my word, but there is a lesson here. Unquestionably, words are uncommonly powerful and intensely essential to society. Without them and their essence human kind would be as cave man, communicating with grunts and hand signals. Worst of all, there would be no Bible, resulting in an acute deficiency of God's basic requirements for social living.

But the Almighty has given us His holy oracles to instruct in the ways of peace and life—and a mind to comprehend and apply the words. Furthermore, God's fundamental prerequisite is this, "He hath shown thee, O man, What is good; and what doth the Lord require of thee but to do justly, and to love mercy, and to walk humbly with thy God" (Micha 6:8).

Clearly, the accent is on four articulate symbols—justice, love, mercy and humility. And I feel God would say to you about them, by all means avoid frivolous stunts like Ole Joe's misuse of redundant. But like him have a love affair with these fabulous words of life, and be truly redundant with them. Recite them over and over—be at-one with them—employ them—and note the change in your life and those about you. You won't be disappointed.

DOES GOD SMOKE

How exciting it was to me to visit the family farm and watch the mule pull the plow—turning the soil over in long gray wakes, and hearing the plowman call out to the animal—"Haw!" (meaning turn left.) "Gee!" (turn right) "Whoa, boy—back up—now, giddyup." It was simply fascinating.

Wow, I wanted to do that, but the fella said I was too little and my Pa might not like it. Then he paused a moment—wiped the sweat off his face and neck and said, "on the other hand, boy, if you'll pick me up a bunch of cigarette butts off the streets in town I'll give you a shot at it."

Undiscerning, I asked why he didn't buy his own smokes. "Hard times," he replied. "No money—it's the depression … or ain't you heard?"

But for some coveted tilling time, though, I happily delivered a paper sack stuffed with unsmoked remains off the sidewalks when I returned. On first sight, the young man eagerly removed the paper from the stubs and mixed the contents in an empty coffee can. Then he loaded some in his corn cob pipe and lit up. I have never seen anyone become so suddenly relaxed. In return for my favor he let me hold the plow handles for about a hundred feet.

Back in town I did some serious thinking. If smoking can make a person feel that good I must be missing out on something extra worthwhile. By all means I must find out for myself.

Opportunity soon walked in. My uncle smoked long, fat cigars from Cuba. He dropped by and conveniently left a lengthy stogie in a saucer on the table. Before Mama could throw it out I took it—got a kitchen match and crawled under the drug store and lit up.

The first pull sort of waved pleasantly in my head. Then another puff. Man O Man, I never felt so relaxed. No wonder the farm boy wanted the street tobacco.

Flushed with light heartedness and well being I sat there in semi dark-
ness blowing smoke and thumping ashes like the grownups. I mimicked
my uncle by clinching the cigar tightly in my teeth while talking. Finally, I
finished the charming thing down to my lips.

Then I crawled out. My first encounter with the creator's cosmos was
the stench of fresh air and the bright sunlight on my face. Instantly, my
will to live vanished.

My liver rolled over and sat up promptly, and spoke harshly to my body
with unbridled quakes—nauseating debilitations and a rapid surge of my
inner contents to the mouth.

On this plateau, reality, time and movement became painfully mud-
dled. Eventually, though, I found myself in front of Dad's store getting
into the cab of his truck. My head fell out the window with no strength to
lift it. A man came over and picked up my face and my eyes fell back like a
toy doll's.

"O, Lord," he said, and rushed into the store.

Immediately, Dad and Mama appeared. The next thing I knew my
father was holding me—shaking me and frantically calling my name and
blowing his breath into my pallid countenance. Mama was hysterical—crying and wringing her hands.

In little time I was home in bed. The family doctor was sitting by me
while someone wiped my lifeless visage with a damp cloth. The physician
touched my chest in several places with his stethoscope and pressed my
stomach with his fingers.

Fortunately, Dad couldn't smell tobacco because of an ancient nose
injury, and Mama was too distraught to sense anything. Not so the medicine man. He was down close to me and he began to sniff.

"Blow your breath in my face, boy," he whispered. I wouldn't do it. He
pinched me hard and said, "Blow!" I did, and his nose crinkled as his lips
pursed tightly together.

Pushing his chair back he turned to my parents and told them not to
worry about me. Such sudden illnesses were fairly common among young
boys and I should fully recover in an hour or so.

Surprisingly, he didn't tell on me. But he bent over me, worrisomely close, and quietly said, "Little boy, go and sin no more lest a worse thing come upon thee the next time you pull such a stunt."

But despite his good advice I did not comply with the practitioner's sound counsel. Fact is, by the time I was twenty-five I was hopelessly addicted, puffing three packs of cigarettes a day.

In addition, my body and clothes reeked of tobacco. I got no rest at night for coughing; I was short of breath and couldn't smell a thing—good or bad. My blood pressure soared. The simple act of eating, drinking or saying hello, called for a smoke. Indeed, as my boyhood G.P. had foretold, a worse thing had come upon me and I had no force over it.

Then, in an extraordinary fashion a higher power came to my rescue. Early on, I had disciplined myself to image the Christ on His cross when conversing with God. Oddly enough, while quietly reflecting on things spiritual one night there came to my apperception a dissimilar depiction in my prayer mode, and without thinking I asked, "Does God Smoke?"

His body and marred head sagged graphically in death as the crucifix shows. But something horribly new was added; for clearly visible in his lips was a smoking cigarette. Needless to say, the vision set me back, but from that day on—every time I spoke to my Creator a lighted smoke appeared in His mouth.

In all honesty, that semblance was my turning point. I laid tobacco aside—never to touch again. My health returned, and the disturbing paradox stopped also.

God helped me free myself from the nicotine bondage—saved my life and gave me self-reliance. However, I might add, the Lord's method of aid to persons are varied and many. His way with you may not be as His manner with me. But He will be to you what you need and what is appropriate for your own personality.

Surely, He will help you release yourself from tobacco's shackles if sincerely asked and heeded. So take these words of His to heart.

"I will strengthen thee; yea, I will help thee; yea, I will uphold thee with the right hand of my righteousness" (Isa. 41:10).

MAKING CHANGE

By any measure, store clerks are honest—hard working persons. But rare, indeed, is the super market cashier who makes change correctly nowadays.

A case in point, at the checkout counter I pull my billfold from my hip pocket with my left hand and hold the wallet that way while the purchases beep over the computer. I extract some currency with my right hand and pay the cashier way—thus freeing my right palm to receive the change.

If properly executed, the silver and four pennies are first laid in the empty hand—then the bills. For all practical purposes, this well-grounded practice has been utilized in retail stores since creation so a customer may—with ease—put the returned paper money in his billfold first—then the coins into his pocket with grace and aplomb.

This approach, by any standard, is by far the best way. But it all depends on how the funds are deposited in the palm.

Corporate intelligentsia, though, has insensitively tossed this tried-and-true method aside and trains their money changers to trash consumer convenience so they can happily complicate shopping life.

Predictably, their flawed enlightenment runs along this line. Instead of the coins the bills are placed in my hand first. Next, an eighteen inch sales slip is plopped on top of that. Then heaped precariously on the lengthy receipt is a pile of silver and copper.

Now what am I to do? Both my hands are full—billfold in the left—money in the right—with no control over the coins. I try desperately to manage but all the metal money slides off and rolls helter-skelter around people's feet.

My next move, of course, is to mumble some inappropriate sounds—grit my teeth, and lay everything in both hands on the counter and retrieve my scattered change while holding up ten impatient shoppers.

Unsettled, I scramble around the floor snatching up as much rolling money as I can and stuff wallet, bills and coins, unarranged, into my pockets. My next move is to get the heck out of there.

Please, Mr. Storeboss, try the old fashioned way one more time. It can save America's sanity.

Clearly, some things should change, albeit, others definitely need not. The first time I heard obscene language at the movies was 1940. It was the "D" word said by Clark Gable in "Gone With The Wind." Suddenly, something was different—something lost.

It was seemingly harmless at the time, but the deviation gained momentum. It didn't eventually fade away or level off—it got worse and spread abroad. Today, a family can't comfortably watch a movie for the inordinate gutter words flushing from the mouths of actors.

I can adjust and cope with the new modes of super store technology, but not this present prurient, topsy-turvy epoch of human history. Undeniably, the so-called new morality is a total failure. The reason: flawed thinking and wrong behavior. The remedy: a transformed mind and decent conduct.

How can a person's destructive direction be rerouted? It's all in the human cognition. Fortunately, providence has provided humankind this formula to heal itself.

"Whatever things are true, whatever things are honest, whatever things are just, whatever things are pure, whatever things are lovely, whatever things are of good report, if there be any virtue, and if there be any praise, think on these things" (Phil 4:8).

By all means, live by these precepts or your life may spin around underfoot, out of control, like my spilled coins.

TRAFFIC LIGHTS

I've discovered that if your natural inclination borders on impatience, a steady diet of red traffic lights will surely push you hypersensitivities to the breaking point, particularly if you're in a hurry.

I am, by a disposition, an impatient person. I simply don't like to wait. In fact, it matters little whether I'm pressed for time or not—I just don't like to be hindered. There runs within me a restless current that demands that I rush ... even if it's unnecessary. Furthermore, after giving considerable thought to my inherent hurriedness I also found that a prolonged lack of patience can make you do and think weird things. "Quite frankly, weird might be a gross understatement.

Few, I'm sure, have heard of the great traffic light conspiracy against me. Of course, you haven't, because it was only recently I became decidedly convinced after catching every red traffic light on a thousand consecutive trips—that those three and four-eye contraptions hanging over intersections and crossroads are alive and have minds of their own. Not only that, but they communicate with each other from Florida to Canada—from the Atlantic to the Pacific, and actually possess the human aptitude to like or dislike persons. What's more, they know you and where you and your car are at all times.

So, by careful observation and some super sleuthing, I concluded correctly that they are out to get some of us. By this, I mean that if you happen to be in their good graces, you get the green—if not, you get the red, every time. I, like most of you, am not in their good favor. They don't like me and I don't like them. Well, the truth is, I hate them.

A lot of things I am, but a dum-dum, I'm not. When I realized what those traffic lights were doing to me, I resolved to get even. Furthermore, I lay awake nights devising schemes to outwit them. My wife, bless her heart, told me to give it a rest ... that I was getting impossible to live with, let alone ride with. Moreover, she advised me to just relax and roll with the traffic before we both have a breakdown. What difference does another minute or two make? Phooey, I thought. Little she knows, I'm in a full scale vendetta with those nasty lights and I aim to win, breakdown or not. Yes, I want to feel revenge's sweetness in my soul.

My initial plan of action was to outwit a hateful old traffic light I stop for each morning and each evening. Predictably, it saw me coming and turned red. Oh, how I hated that red signal. I told a fellow sufferer that I had never in my life caught a green on that wicked light. He said he hasn't either and had quit going that way years ago, and that I ought to do the same. But I was not to be outdone. Some way, some how, I was going to get a good clean green on arrival at that light. I wasn't going another way. No, never. Day and night I visualized the joy of precious victory in my bones.

So I put my stratagem into action. First, I simply tried to sneak up and zip through while it was still green. I failed. Next, I used the element of surprise by quickly turning off a side street into it. Foiled again—stupid light. I took a whack at wreaking its timing by delaying my departure. Another defeat. Six months passed and that light said "gotcha" every time. Finally, under much stress, loss of weight, threats of divorce, and talking flapdoodle nonsense, I gave up, surrendered—waved the white flag. It was a no win agenda. So you see, extreme impatience can make a nervous nut out of you and me and cause us to think and do bizarre things. Whew!

Obviously, most of what is written here is made up. Most, but not all. However, it all has to do with acquiring patience and the Bible has a lot to say about that. Jesus speaks of your soul as your most priceless possession. "In your patience, possess ye your soul," he said (Luke 21:19). Of course, in one's overactive impatience, there is little control over anything because mingled with that restless spirit is intolerance, anger, fussiness, and self inflicted distresses. The attitude of negativism prevails in your personality and you bring gloom to yourself and all those near you.

But all that can be changed. Do what I've begun to do—reluctantly at first—but relax—roll with the traffic—strive to rejoice when the light is red; it simply provides time for you to look up and say, "Praise God."

Then, in your patience possess ye your cool. Patience is a divine quality that can be yours, but how do we get it? It's like John Wesley's formula for obtaining faith—practice it until you have it, and may your good Lord give you patience in your tribulation and travels on this planet.

STATE TROOPERS

If you've ever been stopped by a state highway patrolman, you know first hand how unsettling the experience is. There you are sitting comfortably behind the steering wheel—minding your own business—abiding by the laws of the road, you think. Then suddenly from nowhere there appears in your mirror a distinctly marked car flicking those dreadful blue lights right behind you. Instantly a thousand tributaries of anxiety spring to life and race through your body, soul and spirit, causing arms, hands and legs to shake and tremble as you ever so timidly pull over to the side of the road.

When on the job, state troopers have no smile muscles or humor nerves in their faces. Consequently, their visage appears rock hard and stern. They utter words that resound with authority and their first unsympathetic sentence to the frightful victim is, "Let me see your driver's license, registration certificate and insurance card." Uneasiness discomfits you as your nervous fingers fumble through your wallet or purse while you desperately try to figure out where the registration certificate is.

Once I had a state trooper and his family as members of my church. We soon became good friends, even though it was common knowledge that he would even stop and ticket his wife, mother or children if they violated state traffic laws. I surmised I would be no exception.

But surely, I thought, somewhere beneath that stony exterior of his there must be a bubbling fountain of mercy and compassion. With that in mind, I asked my trooper friend one day, "Now, hypothetically speaking, let's say a pretty young lady was inadvertently breaking the speed limit and you pulled her over—but she sobbed and pleaded with you not to giver her a ticket, and reeled off all manner of high quality excuses—what would you actually do?" My trooper friend thought for a minute and replied. "Oh, I would certainly listen to every word she had to say—and then I would give her a ticket." Well, so much for law and grace.

I have, indeed, suffered the experience of being pulled over twice by the highway patrol over the last twenty years, I think. The first time was for a broken tail light. The next time was on a county road where no state trooper was supposed to be.

It was spring and my wife and I were happily driving along focusing all our attention on the glorious road-side flowers—honey suckle ladened fences and green leafy trees. We were feasting or eyes on God's creation and commenting on some special bit of scenery utterly unaware we were driving all over the road. But, who cared? There was not a car in sight, that is, except for the one in my mirror flashing those awful lights. Where in the world did he come from?

"What are you drinking buddy?" the trooper asked. "You've been wobbling all over the road for miles." And with silent prayer, accompanied with great trepidation, I graciously explained to him that I was not drinking—that I was a United Methodist minister—and all my wife and I were doing was admiring the fantastically beautiful scenery.

None of this, though, changed his uniformed demeanor one iota. He took my license and credentials back to his car. In a few minutes he was back. Fortunately, I had a safe driver's license, so it was only a warning this time. But, next time? Whew! I ventured to insert some humor into his austerity by asking him jokingly to tell my wife to stop talking and showing me things so I could drive straight. No response. Law is law.

Law and grace come to mind at this point. The letter of the law can't be consistently twisted, bent or compromised. Ultimately, it can only be broken. But who can keep every law in the land? And, who even knows all the laws to be obeyed? The Old Testament has five books with hundreds of laws to be adhered to, conveyed with dire consequences for those who transgress its rules. If any person was able to keep God's laws absolutely—that person would be without sin and perfect.

But except for Jesus there has never existed a sinless person on this planet. Jesus alone kept the law. And this same Jesus knows how fallible and fickle we people are. He knew God's laws would condemn and put us all to death and so he moved ahead of the law and gave us mercy and grace and forgiveness. He took the ticket of our violations, faced the judge and paid the price.

Jesus is always at the right hand of power making intercession for our trespasses. Ours is to speak to him daily that we be forgiven for our sins. And when we meet Him face to face we will need no price in our hands to pay out. We simply cling to the cross.

Without Jesus we will be judged by God's law and that will be worse than seeing flashing lights and facing a state trooper.

BEFORE ASPIRIN AND SOME OTHER THINGS

Quite frankly, I feel it next to impossible for people in today's world to envisage what life was like before the emergence of twentieth century medicines.

Take for example the aspirin tablet. In these modern times, those little round white pellets are universally touted as containing counteragent powers to prevent heart attacks, strokes and certain kinds of cancer. Wow! That's great news to me because, like the rest of us, I've gulped down aspirin as far back as I can remember to reduce fever and myriad aches and pains. Accordingly, I was getting additional heath benefits I wasn't even aware of. Great!

There was a time, however, not even a century ago, that the small tablet we thought had been on earth forever existed only on paper. In fact, it did not become the nation's favorite pain killer until well into the 20th century. Taking this into account, I've often wondered how the human species ever survived before aspirin and some other things—seems downright impossible.

Yet humankind did get by without those pills and all the other wonder drugs existing today. That's beyond belief we might think. How could people, by any stretch of the imagination, live and endure without today's amazing physicians and medicines? Well, they did, and a casual reading of "people history" will demonstrate how they managed without the medical technology we have today.

Take a case in point; I have in my possession a rather large, ancient satchel—its leather crumbling with age. It belonged to my late grandmother (1847-1935) on my dad's side. We grandchildren fondly remember her as "Mammy." Occasionally, I find myself rummaging through that old case of hers and once again the history of her world of wilderness homesteading in Florida's panhandle in the second half of the 1800's springs to life. Her's was a land without hospitals, drug stores, and, that's right, no aspirin tablets. The nearest trading store was 20 miles away, traversed by horse, ox, or on foot.

In this rugged environment, Mammy, widowed and with eight children of her own, just naturally fell into the role of homestyle doctor and midwife. She had, by necessity and by her sweet benevolent nature, acquired a superb knowledge of medicinal herbs, healing formulas and their sundry uses.

So knowing a call could come any time for her curative services, she kept her bag, that I now have, stocked with remedies for chills and fevers, pains and ailments and jottings of incantations and written formulas for mixing restorative leaves and roots. Unfortunately, folks in her day knew nothing of what we have today. They simply made do with what they had.

Suppose, for instance, you lived in Mammy's time and your child has a sore throat and fever sores on the lips and gums and did not respond to Mammy's oral medicines. No big deal, because a certain formula of words was waiting in her bag which would surely cure the youngster if these directions were followed precisely.

> "Speak the following and it will certainly help you; Job went through the land holding his staff in his hand, when the Lord did meet him and said to him, Job, what are thou grieved at? Job said, Oh God, why should I not be sad. My throat and my mouth are rotting away. Then said the Lord to Job, 'In yonder valley there is a well which will cure thee,' (name the afflicted person here.) 'and thy mouth and thy throat in the name of God the Father, the Son and the Holy Ghost, Amen.' This prayer must be spoken three times in the mornings and three times in the evenings, and where it reads 'which will cure thee,' you must blow three times in the person's mouth."

Against this backdrop, how did our forbears survive without the miracle tablet? Was it their homespun and superstitious nostrums? Not really.

Long before aspirin, there abode another healer. Without it human existence, indeed would have been intensely difficult, if not impossible.

To characterize it I think of my grandmother—her bag of home remedies at the ready—taking time to offer up a prayer—then riding off into the night on a wilderness trail. Ahead was a sick child, or a life ebbing away—or a new life entering the world or someone in great pain.

What was that overwhelming, comforting palliative of hers that radiated through all night vigils and flowed through her voice and the touch of her hands? It was the greatest healer of them all—love.

And Jesus said, "by this shall all men know that ye are my disciples if ye have love one to another" (John 13:35).

THE VALUE OF
DISCOMFORT

My oldest daughter and her family are into the outdoors and bonfires nowadays. Fortunately, they can happily practice this rustic pastime because they live in the country and have the space and lots of scrap wood to burn.

On weekend days—along about dusk—they, and their kinsmen gather on the banks of their fish pond and build a mammoth fire on the ground. Marshmallows and wieners are roasted on sticks. The kids eat and play while the adults sit on the grass … talk, nibble the food and rivet their eyes on the prancing, red flames.

To tell the truth, I do not know what primordial instinct it is that moves through the veins of my offspring and compels them to abandon the delightful comforts of electric stoves, tables, chairs, screened windows and head for the American outback to build a fire on the dirt and slap at mosquitoes and gnats. But I do know the passion did not originate from their mother and dad.

I never cease to marvel, though, that after thousands of years of Hegelion dialectical struggles to move from the trees and caves into comfortable homes—human kind eagerly chucks it all and happily skips off to the wildwood, and its varmints, to rough it again.

My kids call it a comforting experience. I think it is a primitive, impulse to be uncomfortable.

Peculiar as it seems, however, my wife and I do enjoy riding through the great outdoors and appreciate immensely the wide open environment, and we certainly want to do our part to protect it.

But along about twilight we do not look for campgrounds or a place to boil coffee on an open spit. On the contrary, we look for modern motels to lodge in and fancy restaurants to sup in. Our nature is to gravitate to the comfortable and we have our reasons.

Sometime back my church youth group invited my wife and me to accompany them on a weekend camping trip even if it was only one night. We would sleep in tents and cook our food on an open fire on the turf. It would be loads of fun. We didn't want to go.

But so intense did the kids prevail upon us to join them in their longing to be uncomfortable that we wisely surmised it best to go along. Otherwise, we would forever be loathsome worms in their sight and snubbers of God's resplendent creation. We went.

No need, our young folks ardently assured us—to fret over sleeping arrangements and cooking. They would attend to that. But just prior to our arrival the campsite had sustained a gully-washer rainstorm. In effect, there was a troublesome message in that down pour for my spouse and me.

Foremost, it told us there was no dry wood to burn to make hot coffee. That little inconvenience didn't bother the young folks at all—they drink Pepsi.

Not so for my wife and me. We gulp coffee—lots of it. We don't know who we are until we've had our Maxwell House. In fact, the big daddy of all miseries is to not have coffee. Consequently, we agonized the night suffering acute caffeine withdrawals and tremors.

I slept in the tent with the boys. There was one cot with a tiny couch pillow, a blanket and nine sleeping bags. The cot was for me. I noticed right away there was a support rod across the middle of my bunk and knew it would play havoc with my back.

"Boys," I said, "I'll just fold the cot and sleep on the ground with you."

Nothing doing, they quickly pined. The cot was brought especially for me—and besides they would never, ever allow their pastor to sleep on the ground … never.

Under this circumstance what could I do? I stifled my displeasure and with much vexation groaning inside I mounted my berth—eased my vertebra down on that axle and felt my backbone bend like Robin Hood's bow.

Sleep, indeed, fled from me. The discomfort was simply too much. In desperation I scrunched all of me above the bar except my legs. They pressed heavily across the brace and went to sleep right away.

Furthermore, about 2:00a.m., a family of ill-mannered raccoons invaded our food supplies and stridently wrought utter bedlam. Rest was impossible after that.

At first light we thanked our young hosts for an exciting evening—said good-bye—and sped away like homing pigeons to Beulah's Land of Comfort.

But later, to my surprise, I learned that the comfort I loved so much was not how God appraises worth. On the contrary, I discovered there are distinctive benefits when there is discomfort for the Creator. For example, by no means was Jesus complaining when he voiced the words, "the foxes have holes, and the birds have nests, but I have no place to rest my head" (Matt. 8:20). Even his disciples, like him, rejoiced when life took on undue hardships for Jehovah's course. They knew the value of discomfort. Why that attitude?

Some things come to mind. Let's say you have adamantly stood on the side of God amidst ridicule and pressure. Or gone out of the way to do acts of kindness. Possibly you have made a monetary sacrifice for a good cause. The list is unlimited to be uncomfortable.

Whatever, something notable happens within and the Most High gives you a keen feeling of rightness. There is an absence of anxiety and the heart is filled with well-being and encouragement. Furthermore, the reality of God is heightened in the mind … as it was with those early Christians.

You may not fully sense it at the time but you have connected with your Maker. You have his attention which is your basic need. Now, two lines of communication are open wide to you … yours to God and his to you.

In truth, there is an open channel to Paradise for you—and if allowed, through it comes peace of mind, strength, assurance and every benefit of His promises. Then there is that quiet inner voice that says to you, "be strong, yea, be strong, you can handle it." And you can. You can face life with all its discomforts and prevail. You have God.

DO PETS GO TO HEAVEN?

I'm asked, on occasion, if I believe there is an after life for animals. I know the inquiry is not meant to be facetious because I personally am intensely cognizant of the bond of love that can exist between pet and owner.

There are no pat answers in this area—and the scriptures doesn't deal with definite specifics concerning the future life of the animal kingdom—except, of course, the human species. But who can know what God will do with all the living things He has brought into existence?

And who can second guess the mind of the Creator? His ways are beyond human kind's perception. In Him love is all inclusive, unfailing and eternal; it encompasses far more than mere mortals can ever imagine.

So, if you have an affinity with your beloved animal you know that sort of affection cannot be confined only to creatures like yourself, even though your soul has more value than all flora and fauna. Indeed, how can love be so tenderly consuming and eternal if this is not so?

The light of the world speaks lovingly of sheep and lambs, fowl and fish. The dove represents the presence of Deity. And when Christ returns, He and the armies of heaven will be riding magnificent white horses. Even in the beginning when God evaluated His handiwork—all of it, His delight was expressed in these words, "Very good."

And, too, the apostle brings to mind that the anxious longing of all the earth, which includes all animals and plants, waits eagerly for Adam's curse to be lifted and paradise to begin again (Romans 8:18-22).

I'm sure most, like me, have experienced some mesmerizing scenes in our Maker's incomparable craftsmanship; sights like a buck on a distant hill with his rack of antlers lifted high and his doe grazing nearby—or pelicans crash diving into the water after fish. When I behold such serendipities, the image I am created in, whispers, "very good."

When my wife and I visit our children in Central Florida we travel on 301 South. That route takes us through a little town where I served my first church, as minister, many years ago. We can see the parsonage and the shade trees in the back yard from the highway. Those trees are special to us because the bones of our little dog "Snoopy" rests in the earth beneath their branches.

I loved Snoopy to pieces and think of her often. Fondly, I recall that it was next to impossible to do my sit-ups when she was around. The little thing wanted to stand on my chest and look me in the face. And she just had to sit with me in my rocking chair when I read the paper. Every morning when we let her out she first ran to a particular tree looking for a squirrel to chase. Naturally, her many trips beat a tiny path between back porch and tree.

One morning she bolted out the front door and across the street following our son to school and was hit by a car. Some neighbors buried her for us and we mourned our loss.

Each passing day after that I sadly watched Snoopy's little trail to the tree fade until it was gone and I understood more so the poignancy of those ancient words, "the wind passes, and it is gone, and the place knows it no more" (Ps. 103:16). And all we are left with is an empty heart and fond memories.

And yet, even now when I think of those precious times with our beloved Snoopy I can feel that quiet, soul soothing voice again, "It was very good."

Will we ever see our little dog again? Will you, someday, see your much loved pet again? All I know to do is to put those things into the hands of a loving God who knows our hearts and needs.

But here are some poetic thoughts from my son-in-law, Ralph Alligood, who, so adroitly, addresses this matter by putting some reassuring words on the lips of that One who is love for pet lovers. God.

Heaven's Pets

Do doggies and kittens go to heaven, was asked of me one day.
And I thought to myself, in my usual way.
Should they, or shouldn't they, be up here with me?
Do you ask that question of all things you see?

Or do you think that heaven's so small,
That there's only room for a few of you all?
I want you to know I've worked heard on this place,
And it's open to all, regardless of race.

But it doesn't end there; it's a wide open gate.
I love things with two legs, four legs and eight.
Do you think heaven would be paradise with no flowers
    around,
Or rainbows or butterflies or birds that abound?

I think about all the things you hold dear,
And everything that adds to your short life here.
And I think it a shame to exclude any part,
Of the things you hold so near to your heart.

And that goes double for your four-legged friends,
Who has your affection to the living end.
So if there's a choice place in heaven's home,
It's for your doggies and kittens to romp and roam.

CALL THE PRO

Yes, I'm convinced—and rightly so—that certain persons—with no effort at all, are endowed, at birth, with natural know-how in particular areas of craftsmanship.

I refer to those, otherwise, ordinary guys, that are gifted with exceptional skills at repairing things mechanical ... specifically, those fellas who can fix most anything devised from metal.

Pliers, screwdrivers, wrenches, nut and bolts are infatuated with those can-do sweethearts and happily submit to every little twist and turn of their nimble hands and fingers.

Not so, with me. Chances are I was unloading stock feed at logging sheds when competence at working with metallic things was passed out. To underscore, I have a graphic recall of one experience that will bear this out.

My wife and I—with little circumspection—attempted to do some plumbing work beneath the lavatory in our bathroom one evening. Our restroom was simple and plain. The pipes were exposed with no cover or cabinets built around them.

And, for no practical purpose—there was, smack-dab, in the middle of the duct that came out of the floor and conveyed water to the sink a joint, coupled together with flange and washer and bolted on both sides.

That small redundancy was okay except for the exasperating little defect in the conduit's half juncture. It leaked. In fact, the seepage had become so accelerated my wife kept towels spread beneath it at all times to soak up the water. Indeed, her daily refrain to me was, "I can't stand it any more. When are you going to fix that pipe?"

But calling a plumber cost money, and extracurricular cash at our house was extraordinary scarce. So I kept putting it off hoping my wife would accept the reality that some tribulation was simply a part of life. No such luck, though, she rejected that philosophy flat out, and prevailed upon me so fervently to do something until I finally took a look at her pesky problem.

"Ah, shoot," I said to my dear one. "All that thing needs is a new washer. I'll pick one up after work tomorrow and get that nuisance out of your hair."

The technology used to turn water off at our house was at the meter in the yard. Unfortunately, a special tool was required for that job. Guess what—I didn't have one—but that didn't deter me.

First, I applied the pliers—them the hammer, screwdriver, pecan cracker and every wrench I could find, but couldn't get the water off. It was then, however, a brilliant idea lit up my mind.

I said to my wife, "You know, that's a little pipe and a small washer. If you're game we could have some towels and the mop ready. I could unbolt the coupling … For sure, a little water will escape, but, so what, we have the towels.

"Then, I could slip the old washer out—slide the new one in and bolt it together in no time. This way we won't have to call a professional and pay out good money."

For reasons unknown my wife went along with my innovative proposal. So, undaunted as Jack shinnying up the bean stalk, I proceeded. I employed the pliers. One bolt out, one to go.

With the feel of triumph in my bones I clinched my new washer in my teeth for quick access and turned the second bolt—then another slow, careful turn.

It was sudden. Like a rifle shot, the loosened washer swung out of its hinge sending a stream of water blasting forth with the force of a wide open fire hose in my face.

I fell back—"Towels! Towels!" I squealed, and my wife came a running—then back for more … finally, all of them and the wash cloths too.

The bathroom was a rising lake and the deluge rapidly poured out the door into the hall floating the throw rug into the living room. But with frenzied prayer, supplication, repentance and drenched body I managed to swing the old rapidly fluttering washer back into place and stem the wild flow—somewhat.

And so, with reddish visage and droopy demeanor I stammered to the plumber what had happened. His response was leg slapping, uncontrollable laughter.

In summation—I don't do plumber's work any more. I do the prudent thing. I call the pro.

With that in mind, let's examine this adventure from another perspective. If exterior devices, like my water pipe, can become impaired and in dire need of professional help, so likewise can the inner person.

It is common knowledge, for example, that there has never been so much stress, anxiety, depression, hopelessness, ad infinitum as experienced in today's society.

There are specialists, without question, who offer excellent clinical counsel and treatments for troubled minds and emotional anguish. Unfortunately, however, their services can be financially out of reach for multitudes and the bad time-fiddle inside plays on.

But into this vexation of the soul comes the master with exciting news because there is free therapy for everyone. However, to receive this costless regimen of pause, you must begin seriously seeking a spiritual rest unlike any corporeal relaxation and well being ever felt.

Scripture describes this respite as rest for body, soul and heart. (Soul and heart are, many times, used interchangeable in scripture). Current speech would define this tranquil as discovering rest and peace for body, mind and emotions.

And how do you do a rest that captures that ever evasive peace of mind and self restoration. First, listen carefully to the Great Physician's instructions, "Come unto me, all ye that labor and are heavy laden, and I will give you rest ... learn of me ... and ye shall find rest unto your souls" (Matt. 11:28-30).

Come, learn and find are the key works in this divine prescription. Their principal design is to come to a private place. Be still and quiet with your cognition focused on your invisible, loving Creator. Let your muscles and your head relax until your tension and heartbeat subsides. You can feel it happening.

Then, by all means, read some Bible. The Gospel of John is a good place to start. Pray some, forgive a lot, meditate some—get in touch with yourself and God and accept His promise that peace and joy are your rightful heritage ... given to you by your Maker. This is to be done daily, even if you have only five or ten minutes to spare.

And don't stop there. Continue throughout the day by saying periodically, "Thank you, Lord," or, "Praise God," or whatever is appropriate for you. Such practice does something beautiful for your whole being. For one thing, it keeps you tuned into the power of the universe. And not only that, the Lord's channel is wide open to you also.

So why not call upon Jesus, the divine Pro. Let Him help you with your hurt and despair and what seems impossible. It will do you good. Otherwise, you could get frequent, unwanted showers by striving to replace flawed washers in your soul. Glory.

THAT'S LIFE, PAPA

At the time my wife and I had four little granddaughters. They were prized darlings of great price … The delight of our lives.

On the downside, though, there existed some minor problems with each one's relationship with their old—exceptionally generous grandpa—me, of course—yours truly.

For example, when one got near me I picked the child up—nuzzled it under the chin with my nose and tenderly cooed, "Papa's little girl." But such fondness on my part became somewhat disheartening at times because my youngster, all too often, responded to my loving gestures by saying, "No, Papa, I'm Grandma's little girl."

I got a little perturbed, indeed, at those constant put-downs. After all, I did a lot for my grandkids. Simply put, I honestly felt I wasn't getting the affection and affirmation due an aging, lovable Gramps who gave his tots whatever they wanted. So I decided I wasn't going to be mishandled any more by my wee progenies. There, I said it, and I stand by it.

For one thing their attention span, to say the least, wasn't acclimatized to entertain good sage advice from me, for long. A case in point was when I told my dear ones that if anyone inquired as to where they got their good looks to always say they were made in the spitting image of their grandpa.

Eventually, a school teacher did ask one where all her prettiness came from. Her response wasn't quite right. "I was made in the image of my spittin' grandpa," she proudly proclaimed to her school mistress.

Another time they were all at my home playing squealing and running from room to room. I sat by the door trying to grab one to hug as they flew by, but they all managed to stay just out of reach. Not to be outdone, though, I lunged at them and caught my five-year old by the arm. She struggled to break loose to continue her playing but with eyes blazing I shouted, "Stop! I want to talk to you right now—here, sit in that chair, there!"

Startled, my tiny one obeyed immediately and plopped down in the chair with chin in hand and stared at me with her big brown eyes, waiting to hear what the old man had to say.

"Look," I said, "I'm your grandpa—your own flesh and blood—do you understand that?" She shrugged her little shoulders.

"Well, let me ask you something," I continued. "Do you know from whence all your blessings flow? They come from me, that's who. Where in heavens name do your think the potato chips, candy, toys and Pepsi come from?"

"Grandma."

"No, no, no, it's me, your papa that gets all these things for you … me, me, me, can't you get that into your pretty head?"

With unblinking eyes she squinched her shoulders again.

"Listen," I whined. "I don't think I'm getting the attention and consideration due me from you guys. And besides, I need more hugs and kisses from my grandkids—it's the least you could do. Now, what do you think of that?"

With that said, my sweet thing sat there for a few moments—chin still nestled in her hand—seemingly in deep thought. Then she answered as profoundly as any old scholar could speak as she hopped out the chair. "Well, Papa, sorry, but that's life." And she scampered off to play. Befuddled, I sat in wood-faced silence a long time pondering the depths of that experience.

More than all other desires, I delight most being in the presence of my children's children. Their worth to me is more than solid gold a million times over … even more than the universe. And the words I want to hear from them often is "Papa, I love you."

Now, by the same token God is much like a loving grandfather. He allows humans to live their own lives—take Him for granted, and even ignore Him. Yet His love for people is never diminished.

But like an old grandfather, the Creator also needs a person's love expressed to Him. Indeed, when my children and grandchildren convey their affection my way my heart soars and I feel a warmness past under-standing. In like manner, so does your Father in heaven when you disclose your love for Him.

One of the best ways I know to express adoration to God is to simply tell Him. That's life—and life abundantly. Give it a try.

THE GREAT BLUE HERON

Cleverly camouflaged the trap hung over a narrow, laid-back rivulet ... widening and quietly ebbing into my fish pond. For sure—I'd never seen anything like this before.

But, there it was ... dangling unnoticed, until now, from a mossy Cypress branch.

The snare was a thin wire cable with a large un-baited steel hook attached. From all appearances it was there to bag an alligator.

"Poachers," I thought. Hey, what's going on here?" And, on top of that, what to do?

Well, I would simply bring my wire cutters the next day on my morning walk—and dismantle this unsettling device.

But, I was too late. On the morrow the hidden contraption had caught ... not an alligator but a Great Blue Heron.

The sight was, indeed, sudden and jolting. The big bird ... hooked under the first joint of his left wing—sagged motionless on the wire. His heavy body stretched out like a wet beach towel fastened at one corner.

Grim as the egregious scene was, I could only marvel at how this wise old fowl of air and water could manage to fall victim to makers of gator traps.

At this point I was slowly assuming what probably happened to put the heron in such jeopardy.

I surmised the hapless beauty ... his slender legs straight down in landing mode—wings spread nearly six feet—a natural crink in his elongated neck—gracefully gliding in to alight in the shallows at the water's edge.

But mindless of the hidden danger, his wing unwittingly swiped the hook, causing it to penetrate deep into his left pinion.

No doubt the unfortunate wader panicked.

I imagined wild confusion breaking in—his free wing flapping hysterically while his hefty body fiercely thrashed about to free himself. But, the taut hook only sliced further into bone.

Now, strength depleted, the captive creature hung limp and still. The pain of the embedded hook had likely traumatized his body and wrenched his wing upward. His feet inept—floated in the water. He could barely hold his wobbly head up. By all accounts he was gator bait.

There was no time to dawdle. If the big blue was to live he must be freed at once—because alligators, inherently, can detect the slightest commotion in the water and move quickly to its source. The big blue could be a gator's delicacy.

It wasn't, in fact, unusual for an occasional alligator to migrate from an adjacent pond down stream (about a hundred yards) to my pool—along with turtles and snakes. For some feathered animals, life could be deadly.

On the opposite side of my modest lagoon a great pine tree had recently blown down and lay along the water's edge. The needles on the branches were still green and thick.

My greatest impediment, though, would be the mud bar just beneath the water's surface—two feet thick and ringing the entire pond. My only in-hand asset was my staff.

This dense sediment collecting at the stream's convergence with my pool made wading virtually impossible. But, wade I must if the creature was to survive.

Then, again, I had no idea what the bird's temperament might be. After all, he was a wild animal, and big. His beak was like a spear.

I had heard of Blue's snapping up minnows off the seat of an aluminum boat … leaving little ice-pick dents with each peck. What could he do to my eyes and face?

Nevertheless, I hastily devised a plan. I pulled off my Reeboks and socks—turned up my pants legs above my knees—and with staff in hand I cautiously stepped into the spillway.

At once I sank to my hips in dark water and leg-clutching muck. It was as I expected … exceedingly difficult to lift a foot and take a step.

But that I did—one painfully, slow, sucking step after another until I was right next to my feathered fowl.

For balance I pushed my staff down to firmer ground. When it held I gently leaned against it and reached for the bird.

It was then—just a quick glimpse from the corner of my eye ... something upstream moved. Something resembling a slab of tire retread—could be a big turtle or even a gator. Whatever, the sight added urgency to my task.

"Easy, boy," I said gently.

With my right hand I opened his left wing and began the daunting task of removing the hook.

While I toiled, the wader's head dropped down and he stared me straight in the face. His sharp beak just inches away.

"My friend," I pleaded. "What ever you do, please don't peck me."

To my surprise the great bird didn't struggle, flinch or make a sound. His unfaltering cooperation and endurance was nothing less than remarkable as I worked at the hook.

I took another flash survey upstream. The retread was much closer.

"Oh, boy," it was indeed a gator. I could make him out now. I worked frantically.

Again, I spoke softly to my feathered victim. "See what you got me into. I bet you don't appreciate, at all, what I'm doing for you—do you?"

No answer, "Dumb bird."

I took another hasty look for the gator. He had disappeared. I guessed he was closing in fast. His target—my Great Blue Heron.

At last the hook loosened. Another fast peek.

The movement of the water told me the reptile was just beneath the surface rapidly approaching the bird and me. The hook broke free.

Desperate, I lifted the weighty bird high over my head with both hands—like a basketball—and gave my best shot to toss him across the confluence toward the pine laying along the shore. The heron came up short and splashed just shy of the fallen tree.

In the process I felt the water rush against my belly as the alligator passed in pursuit of his prey.

The bird—his injured wing open and hanging useless—struggled to get out of the water and into the toppled pine.

I was frantic. "Get out of the water," I yelled over and over.

Just as the bird pulled himself to safety in the tree branches, the water heaved and lapped at the pine boughs. The gator had aborted his quest.

But end of story is not yet. For sure, I was in a hurry to get out of the water. The gator was still in the pond somewhere … with me.

I grasped my staff and began the arduous task of backing out. Finally, I felt the mud's grip give way to solid ground. And then I stepped back on dry earth—relief.

After washing the silt from my feet and legs, I donned my socks and shoes.

For the moment I had done all I could for the heron. When I left my miniature lake, I could see his head and neck—like a periscope—rising above the pine boughs.

Hopefully, he could rest and gain enough strength to feed himself from the pond. I would monitor his condition daily.

My son-in-law has two frisky dogs—ready to chase anything, but unemployed I often take them on my walks. Nevertheless, it soon became apparent it best to leave the canines behind. They would like nothing better than to rout my wounded bird.

But along with his mending the creature began to roam to other ponds in search of food, dragging his injured wing … fair game for the dogs. I wandered if he would ever fly again before he was mauled by the mutts. He, of course, endured many narrow escapes.

Then one day the two dogs caught big blue in the open field on his visit to another pond. In a barking frenzy they went after him.

The bird tried to run but that was virtually impossible with his disabled wing.

However, in spite of his wound he did run. And just as the two howling—leaping animals closed in, the beautiful wader spread his great wings and took flight into the safety of the pond.

I was delighted, to say the least. Under my eyes the mighty fowl improved daily. I teased my friends about my unusual relationship with the Great Blue.

For fun, I even told them my bird tipped his wings when he flew over the house just to say thank you. But, that wasn't so.

I like to think, though, that nature—in its awesome mystery—has a way of letting one know it approves of kindnesses to God's creatures.

One morning I opened the gate to take my walk. There on the ground was this gigantic wing feather from a Great Blue Heron.

Well, how do I feel about this?

I like to think this fowl of air and water broke through the mystery of creation and in his way said to me, "thank you for what you did for me."

I saw the great bird many times after that—his wings spread nearly six feet—his thin legs in landing mode—gracefully gliding into my pond to alight in the shallows at the water's edge.

And in awe, I whisper the words from the Ancient Oracle, "Very good."

In my anxiety I once said to my Blue Heron, "Dumb bird."

I take it back.

MACH VELOCITY

Canoes—traditionally—are narrow boats, piked at both ends, and designed to support two, 145 pound, nimble tribesmen to sit at each end. Indeed, their design is restricted and not intended to sustain a pair of 220 pound greenhorns whose sheer weight, presses the vessel's rim perilously near water level with little or no space to spare.

Like other outdoorsmen, one of the most notable joys of my life is fishing, but far more stimulating is hyperbolizing some of my successful, angling outings to anyone who will listen. I don't usually tell of the unprosperous trips though—too embarrassing. After all, it's more mollifying to stay with the fruitful stories—keeps pride and ego intact.

Nonplus, as it is, I feel compelled to lay bare one of my fishing reveries simply to warn those cumbrous hefties who, like me—live on the edge, and fish from wee canoes.

Previously, my daughter had given me an expensive Stetson to wear in the open sun. I cherished that hat and cocked it on my head proudly on many occasions, fully cognizant how debonair I must look. More to the point, however, I wouldn't even think of wearing my exquisite head piece on pond water—except—that is, on this one particular morning when I forgot my cap.

It was steamy hot on the lake. My son-in-law, Ralph, and I, worked the lily pads and grassy patches along the shore line—catching nothing. We surmised the fish had moved to a deeper, cooler environment. I adjusted my hat to shade my eyes as we paddled out and fished deep.

Happily, we began picking up some crappie and bream. I tossed my line into the depths and paused for my beetle-spin lure to drop near the bottom. Then I reeled in slowly. WHAM! An angry bluegill was on my hook—my line sang as it sliced the surface and bent my rod almost double. Hallelujah! I shouted, as I wound him in.

Indeed, with galloping heart—trembling fingers and pasty mouth I hurriedly repeated the same procedure. But by this time the boat was drifting and I was forced to twist my overweight bulk to the right, causing some intense body strain. I quickly forgot that, though, when I felt the titillating snatch on my line again.

But as I spooled in, the feisty fish decided to cut behind my back adding more painful tension to my spine. Instantly, and awkwardly, I endeavored to swing the rod backward and over my head and comfortably bring my prize in from the left.

As a result, the canoe tipped ominously to the right. I panicked and threw my weight to the left and dipped in some pond. Sudden trepidation seized me as I snapped back to the starboard causing the boat to flip at mach velocity. Ralph and I were in the water.

When I broke the surface my first gratification was seeing my precious Stetson floating nice and level on the water. I quickly placed my left hand over my shirt pocket to save my glasses. With my free hand I retrieved my hat. But an abrupt revelation awakened me to the fact that one can't remain afloat that way. It is virtually impossible to swim from the elbows back.

Simply put, my beloved Stetson received baptism that day along with my damaged ego. And the gorgeous hat lost its splendor and took on the tarnished gray of a floppy head piece—conditioned for an African Safari. Laughter still gushes from Ralph when my repertoire comes up—but I sort of half-grin and suggest talking about something else. Whew!

Sometime back, it was my honor, to participate in the funeral of a dear African-American lady. Her minister gave the principal eulogy and I thought it the most succinct discourse I'd ever heard at such an occasion.

He said he wasn't preaching her funeral for she already done that—and that we are all living our own final tributes as we walk out our days. His admonishment was the uncertainty of each hour with no promise of tomorrow. The Bible assures no one of a long life he counseled. But warns everyone to "be ready to meet your maker" at a moment's notice.

I didn't know I would turn a boat over that day. It happened suddenly—in an instant. Office workers sitting at desks—persons eating at restaurants, children at school, do not know if someone with a deadly weapon will walk in and begin firing. Some employees going to work at the Federal Building in Oklahoma City did not know that day was their last.

Add to this the plane crashes and auto accidents and multitudes of other ways to stop breathing and we see how unpredictable an hour is.

"Be ready," the Preacher informs. "You could be before the judgment in less than a minute. Yea, I say again, be ready."

978-0-595-41608-0
0-595-41608-X